THE MEDICINE-FREE,
ILLNESS-FREE SERIES

DETOXIFICATION THERAPY

Cleanse, Recharge, and Rejuvenate for Vibrant Health

Forest Yin, DAOM, L.Ac.

Ashi Healing Publishing

First Edition: May 2025

Published by Ashi Healing

www.AshiHealing.com

Paperback ISBN: 978-1-967735-12-9

eBook ISBN: 978-1-967735-13-6

Printed in the United States of America

Medical Disclaimer:

This book is for informational purposes only and is not intended as medical advice. The author and publisher assume no responsibility for how the information is used. Readers should consult a healthcare professional before making any health-related decisions.

Foreword

Nature is the origin of life, the origin of healing, and remains a guiding force in human well-being. Long before modern science developed medicine in laboratories, nature provided everything the human body needed to survive, and to sustain life. The food we eat, the herbs we gather, the minerals beneath our feet, and the sun above us are all part of an intelligent and interconnected system that has long nourished and supported the human body.

This truth has been known across cultures for thousands of years, and it is echoed in sacred texts. In the Book of Genesis, the Garden of Eden was described as a paradise where "every tree that is pleasant to the sight and good for food" was made available to humankind (Genesis 2:9). Some scholars believe this refers not only to nourishment, but also to the ability to contribute to human well-being. It becomes even more clear in Ezekiel 47:12: "The fruit thereof shall be for meat, and the leaf thereof for medicine."

Somewhere along the way, modern culture drifted from this wisdom. Many now believe that healing must come through synthetic drugs, surgeries, or man-made interventions, forgetting that the foundation of human health has always been rooted in nature. But what if well-being isn't only about medical breakthroughs, but also about reconnecting with what has always been available to us?

What if the body doesn't need to be forced to function differently, but simply supported, nourished, balanced, and reminded of what it already knows? What if illness is not the enemy, but a signal that we've fallen out of balance, and out of sync with nature?

This is not to dismiss the value of conventional medicine. We are deeply grateful for its life-saving capabilities in emergencies and acute care. But when it comes to supporting long-term vitality and encouraging balance, it may be time to return to the source.

In addition to thousands of years of lived wisdom, modern science is now exploring the potential of many natural approaches. What was once viewed as "alternative" is now increasingly recognized as part of a broader wellness conversation.

This book, and the entire *Medicine-Free, Illness-Free Series*, is rooted in this truth:

Nature not only gave us life. Many believe it holds the power to support our well-being. And many of these natural approaches are now being studied and better understood through science.

Healing is not something we must force or fear. It is something we can encourage, by gently supporting the body, naturally.

Dr. Forest Yin, DAOM, L.Ac.

Author, *The Medicine-Free, Illness-Free Series*

Founder, Ashi Healing and Acupuncture Inc.

Important Disclaimer

The supplements, therapies, and natural approaches discussed in *The Medicine-Free, Illness-Free Series* are intended to support general wellness and the body's natural balance. They are not intended to diagnose, treat, cure, or prevent any disease and have not been evaluated by the U.S. Food and Drug Administration (FDA).

These books are provided for educational purposes only and are not a substitute for professional medical advice, diagnosis, or treatment. Always consult your physician or a licensed healthcare provider before starting any new supplement, therapy, or wellness routine, especially if you are pregnant, nursing, have a medical condition, or are taking medications.

The content in this series is informed by two sources: summaries of available scientific research, presented as "Science-Informed Solution Benefits", and aggregated user feedback, presented as "Customer-Reported Solution Benefits". These are intended to inform and inspire, but they reflect general patterns, not guarantees. Individual results will vary.

The phrase *"Medicine-Free, Illness-Free"* reflects a natural wellness philosophy and is not a medical claim or promise of outcome.

By reading this book, you agree to take full responsibility for your personal health choices and to seek guidance from qualified health professionals when needed.

Contents

Preface

Do you feel like you've tried everything—medications, conventional treatments, even supplements—yet still struggle with fatigue, discomfort, brain fog, or other daily wellness concerns?

If so, you're not alone.

Many people today are turning to nature-based solutions, not as replacements for essential medical care, but as gentle, sustainable ways to support their overall well-being.

The rise in chronic health challenges reflects this shift. According to the CDC, over 60% of U.S. adults live with at least one chronic health condition, and more than 40% manage two or more. More than 40% of school-aged children in the United States are reported to have at least one ongoing wellness concern, rising sharply in recent years.

At the same time, modern habits, nutrient-depleted diets, environmental stressors, and sedentary routines, have created a disconnect between how we live and what the body truly needs to stay resilient. For many, conventional solutions haven't fully addressed these patterns, leaving people still searching for support that feels both effective and sustainable.

That's what *The Medicine-Free, Illness-Free Series* is here to explore.

This series introduces practical, natural options that may help support energy, digestion, sleep, focus, mood, and more, without requiring major lifestyle changes or complicated routines.

It doesn't reject conventional medicine. It expands your toolkit. While modern treatments often focus on managing symptoms in the short term, natural health practices are designed to work more gradually, supporting the body's natural rhythms over time. Many people are rediscovering how ancient practices and modern science can work together, not in opposition, to create a more balanced, resilient life.

The Medicine-Free, Illness-Free Series is built on two foundational pillars:

Science-Informed Solution Benefits: exploring what modern research says about the potential benefits associated with each supplement or therapy

Customer-Reported Solution Benefits: drawn from thousands of real-world user feedback to highlight what people most often experience in practice, including common benefit themes, typical use case patterns, and key user insights.

By combining scientific research with traditional use and real-world user feedback, each volume empowers you to make informed decisions, grounded in both evidence and everyday reality.

Each book in the series focuses on one category of natural therapies. Whether you're exploring Herbal Therapy, Mushroom Therapy, Amino Acid support, Animal Organ Supplements, Grounding, the HOPED Protocol, or detoxification, the goal is the same: to offer trusted solutions that fit easily into your life, simply, naturally, and sustainably.

You don't need to overhaul your lifestyle or commit to an elaborate health plan. You can begin right where you are. Even one small step, a single herb, nutrient, or daily practice, can help you create a rhythm of care that supports your body more naturally over time.

Preface

While no approach guarantees results, many people have found these natural strategies helpful in supporting comfort, energy, focus, and overall vitality. This series was created to help you explore those tools with clarity and confidence, without pressure or complexity.

This volume focuses on Detoxification Therapy, offering practical insight into time-tested ingredients and natural methods that help support the body's detox pathways. You'll learn about each approach through both research and real-world perspectives, so you can decide what feels right for your journey.

Thank you for beginning this exploration.

Let's move forward, one natural step at a time.

The Medicine-Free, Illness-Free Series

The Medicine-Free, Illness-Free Series is your go-to resource for practical, research-informed natural strategies that are easy to apply. Each volume focuses on a single modality or system—herbs, mushrooms, organ supplements, amino acids, grounding, detox, and more—offering clear guidance to help you choose what works best for you.

Together, the 10 books provide a comprehensive yet flexible wellness framework that supports both daily health maintenance and targeted support. Here's a brief overview of what you'll find in each book:

The Medicine-Free, Illness-Free Series: Why Natural Health Is the Future

Explore why millions of people are turning to nature-aligned strategies to support their wellness. This foundational volume introduces the core science and philosophy behind natural approaches to health, and how they may support your sense of balance, vitality, and overall well-being.

The Medicine-Free, Illness-Free Series: Herbal Therapy

Learn how the world's most time-tested plants may support digestion, energy, relaxation, immune strength, and more. Discover practical ways to include them in your routine and how to choose herbs that match your personal needs and constitution.

The Medicine-Free, Illness-Free Series: Mushroom Therapy

Discover the unique compounds found in medicinal mushrooms that may support immunity, cognitive function, and stress resilience. This book explains how to use mushrooms such as Reishi, Lion's Mane, and Cordyceps in a daily supplement.

The Medicine-Free, Illness-Free Series: Animal Organ Therapy

Explore how nutrient-dense organ supplements, like liver, heart, and kidney, may provide highly bioavailable vitamins, minerals, and peptides. Learn how these traditional foods may support foundational wellness in areas like energy, endurance, and metabolic balance.

The Medicine-Free, Illness-Free Series: Amino Acid Therapy

Uncover the role of amino acids, the building blocks of life, in supporting mood, focus, muscle strength, and nervous system health. This volume shows how targeted amino acid support may help restore clarity, resilience, and emotional well-being.

The Medicine-Free, Illness-Free Series: HOPED Protocol

Learn the five foundational nutrient categories—High Fiber, Omega-3s & Antioxidants, Probiotics, Enzymes, and Vitamin D—and how to implement them as a core wellness strategy. HOPED is simple, actionable, and designed for everyday consistency.

The Medicine-Free, Illness-Free Series: Detoxification Therapy

Discover a gentle, nature-based approach to support your body's natural detoxification processes, promote balance, and encourage overall vitality using simple, practical techniques.

The Medicine-Free, Illness-Free Series: Grounding Therapy

Explore the science and practice of grounding (earthing), the natural process of reconnecting with the Earth's electrical field. Learn how this subtle practice may help support nervous system regulation, sleep quality, and emotional balance.

The Medicine-Free, Illness-Free Series: Diet, Lifestyle and Emotional Well-being

While drastic changes are not required, this volume introduces simple habits that promote long-term balance, covering food, movement, sleep, and emotional self-regulation in a way that aligns with the rest of your natural health plan.

The Medicine-Free, Illness-Free Series: Integrative Therapies for Everyday Health

This final volume brings together insights from the entire series, offering user-reported tools to help support everyday wellness goals, such as energy, digestion, sleep, immunity, and emotional resilience. It serves as a cross-reference for applying the therapies in complementary ways, helping you navigate your health journey with clarity and confidence.

Meet Dr. Forest Yin, DAOM, L.Ac.

Professionally known as Forest Yin, my official name is Jie Yin, while also known as 尹明杰 in the Chinese speaking communities.

For most of my professional life, I was known as a high-tech executive, problem-solver, and innovator in information security and technologies. In leadership roles at Oracle, Schwab, and Wells Fargo, I developed and managed advanced security solutions, ensuring stability, efficiency, and high performance in a fast-paced, high-stakes environment.

But after work, I was deeply immersed in another world, the science of natural health.

My journey into Traditional Chinese Medicine (TCM) began in college, when I first studied the *Huang Di Nei Jing (Yellow Emperor's Classic of Internal Medicine)* alongside my Physics degree. While excelling in my tech career, I continued to research, experiment, and apply natural healing principles, seeking ways to optimize health, energy, and resilience, not just for myself, but for those around me.

Recognizing the profound impact of natural medicine on long-term health and performance, I pursued formal training, becoming a Licensed Acupuncturist (L.Ac.) in 2018 and earning my Doctorate in Acupuncture and Oriental Medicine (DAOM) in 2019. Since then, I have supported individuals around the world in improving their vitality, resilience, and sense of well-being through natural methods. This led me to found Ashi Healing and Acupuncture Inc. and become a Professor and Doctoral Advisor at the University of East-West Medicine, where I mentor future practitioners in the art of TCM.

Applying Systems Thinking to Health & Healing

In high-tech, solving problems requires understanding systems, identifying vulnerabilities, and optimizing performance. I apply the same mindset to health. Instead of treating symptoms, I look at the root cause, like debugging a system. Instead of temporary fixes, I focus on long-term balance and resilience, like designing sustainable architecture. Instead of pharmaceutical dependency, I seek efficient, natural approaches that support function and balance gently, without the common side effects associated with conventional options, like optimizing system performance.

While many of my colleagues in the tech and finance industries thrived in their careers, I also saw the toll of chronic stress, burnout, autoimmune conditions, and lifestyle-related illnesses. Like many professionals, they pushed their limits, until their bodies pushed back. This is where natural approaches can make a difference.

A Philosophy Rooted in Balance & Natural Healing

At Ashi Healing, my approach complements conventional care by focusing on identifying underlying imbalances and supporting the body's natural self-regulation through Traditional Chinese Medicine and holistic strategies.

The name "Ashi (阿是)" comes from a fundamental concept in Chinese medicine, that moment of realization when healing feels real. In Chinese, "Ashi" means "Ahh, Yes!", the instant when your body recognizes exactly what it needs. This guiding philosophy shapes everything I do, from acupuncture to natural health solutions.

Through the precise use of Chinese Herbal Medicine and modern whole-food-based natural supplements like herbs and mushrooms, I have helped individuals support their energy and balance naturally, using simple, sustainable tools that complement or reduce the need for pharmaceutical interventions when appropriate.

My mission is simple: to help people pursue wellness and resilience, naturally and sustainably.

Integrating Ancient Wisdom with Modern Innovation

Chinese Herbal Medicine has been refined for thousands of years. But today, we can take it further, combining ancient wisdom with modern research and a strategic, data-driven approach to health optimization.

At Ashi Healing, I personalize each protocol based on the individual's needs, whether it's boosting energy, reducing stress, improving cognitive function, or addressing chronic health concerns. Many of the people I work with are busy professionals seeking practical, time-efficient strategies to support their health without disrupting their demanding schedules.

Looking for More Information and Support

To learn more about my personalized approach to Chinese Herbal Therapy and whole-food-based supplements, visit AshiHealing.com. You'll find additional resources and simple ways to take the next step in your healing journey, whenever you're ready.

And remember, this book is just one part of *The Medicine-Free, Illness-Free Series.* Each volume explores a different pillar of natural healing, from herbs and mushrooms to amino acids, detoxification, and grounding, offering you a complete path to support your balance and well-being through nature-based strategies.

A Science-Backed, Real-World Tested Method

In *The Medicine-Free, Illness-Free Series,* we introduce a unique, structured method for exploring natural supplements, one that blends scientific insight with real-world observations. Rather than relying solely on clinical studies or anecdotal reports, we combine both perspectives to give you a well-rounded, user-friendly understanding of each natural solution.

This balanced approach helps answer the most important questions: What does science suggest about this supplement's potential? What are people actually experiencing when they use it? Which health goals do people turn to it for most often?

Our method reflects a commitment to transparency, education, and practicality, so you can explore these natural options with clarity and confidence.

Our Four-Part Analysis Method

1. Science-Informed Solution Benefits

We begin by reviewing peer-reviewed studies, traditional usage patterns, and emerging scientific literature to understand the possible mechanisms and effects of each supplement. This provides a foundation of what is known, hypothesized, or being actively researched, offering a science-informed perspective to guide your exploration.

2. Customer-Rcported Solution Benefits

We analyze large sets of customer reviews from publicly available platforms to understand how these supplements are being used in daily life. This includes what benefits people say they notice most often and how they describe their experiences.

Our focus is on patterns of what users commonly report, rather than isolated stories. This real-world layer helps connect the theory to practical, everyday outcomes.

3. Use Case Patterns & Feedback Insights

Within the customer-reported section, we highlight:

Use Case Patterns Observed – What kinds of goals or wellness concerns people most commonly use each supplement for.

Feedback Insights – How users describe the impact in their own words, including sentiment, language tone, and satisfaction cues.

Most Reported Benefits – A percentage-based summary showing which benefits are mentioned most often in reviews.

This structured summary lets you see what real people are using the supplement for, and how frequently those benefits are reported.

4. No Brand Promotion—Just Trusted Guidance

This series does not promote specific products or brands. Instead, we offer education and a decision-making framework. For those looking for high-quality sources, recommended supplement types and vetted options are available at AshiHealing.com.

Why This Method Matters

In today's crowded supplement market, it can be hard to separate hype from helpful information. That's why we created this approach, to empower you with insights drawn from scientific research, real-world usage patterns and satisfaction trends, and clear summaries that help you compare options and set expectations

You won't find exaggerated claims or one-size-fits-all solutions here. Instead, you'll find a practical, transparent method that reflects how real people are exploring natural wellness, with science as a guide and personal experience as a reference.

Whether you're considering herbs, mushrooms, amino acids, or other supplements, this method gives you a safe and structured way to learn how others are using these tools, and how they might fit into your own wellness journey.

A Personal Commitment from Dr. Forest Yin

Every approach, strategy, and supplement featured in *The Medicine-Free, Illness-Free Series* has been personally explored. Before sharing any recommendations with clients or readers, I take the time to experience it myself, observing how it affects energy, mood, sleep, digestion, and focus.

This hands-on approach allows me to understand each therapy not just through science, or just through other people's experiences. It adds a personal layer of insight to the research and user-reported feedback that shape this series.

My goal is simple: to help you find natural, sustainable solutions that feel doable, helpful, and aligned with how lasting wellness begins, by reconnecting with your body's own rhythms and innate intelligence.

Cleansing Your Body for Health

Every day, your body is exposed to a surprising number of toxins, many of which are hidden in plain sight. From the air you breathe and the food you eat to the water you drink and the products you apply to your skin, toxic substances gradually accumulate. Industrial pollutants, pesticides, food additives, heavy metals, plastics, mold toxins, and synthetic chemicals all contribute to this invisible but significant burden.

In addition to environmental exposure, lifestyle factors such as poor diet, chronic stress, lack of physical activity, and inadequate sleep can impair your body's natural detoxification systems. Toxins often build up in the liver, kidneys, colon, lymphatic system, and fat cells, slowing elimination and potentially contributing to issues such as persistent fatigue, brain fog, sluggish digestion, bloating, hormonal fluctuations, lowered immune function, skin imbalances, and difficulty maintaining a healthy weight.

The encouraging news is that your body is already equipped with systems designed to detoxify itself. When given the right support, these systems can work efficiently to help restore energy, improve digestion, and enhance overall well-being. Detoxification does not require extreme diets or aggressive cleanses. It is about removing the burdens that interfere with your body's natural balance so it can perform at its best.

This book serves as a practical guide to supporting your body's detox capacity. You will learn about liver detox, colon cleansing, parasite protocols, heavy metal elimination, lymphatic drainage, kidney support, and candida and yeast balancing. Each plays a unique role in helping your body maintain vitality and resilience.

Understanding Detoxification and Its Importance

Detoxification is not a passing trend. It is a vital biological function that supports balance and long-term health. The liver, kidneys, digestive tract, lymphatic system, lungs, and skin all work together to process and eliminate unwanted substances from the body. However, in today's environment, the volume of toxic exposure is often more than these systems can handle alone.

When the detoxification process slows or becomes overwhelmed, toxins can accumulate in tissues and organs. This may contribute to systemic stress, chronic inflammation, and imbalances that affect energy, mood, digestion, immunity, and skin clarity. Fatigue, mental fog, joint stiffness, and other nagging symptoms are often early signs that the body's cleansing systems need additional support.

When properly supported, detoxification helps the body work more efficiently. The liver processes chemicals and metabolic waste, the kidneys filter the blood, the colon eliminates solid waste, and the lymphatic system assists in cellular cleanup. Encouraging these systems to function well may result in clearer thinking, improved digestion, better skin, higher energy levels, and stronger natural defenses.

Detoxification is not something you do once. It is a foundational element of preventive health. By learning how to reduce your exposure and support your body's ability to eliminate waste, you can build resilience, feel better each day, and protect your health over the long term.

The Body's Natural Detox Systems

Before diving into specific detox protocols, it's important to understand how your body is already designed to cleanse and restore itself. Detoxification isn't something you force, it's something you support. Your body works constantly, around the clock, to neutralize and eliminate waste, toxins, and byproducts that accumulate from food, environmental exposure, internal metabolism, and stress. The more we support these systems, the more resilient and energized we become.

Here's a concise overview of the body's major detox systems and their vital roles:

Liver – The Master Filter

The liver is one of the most powerful detoxification organs in the body. It processes everything from food and medications to alcohol and environmental toxins, breaking them down into safer substances that can be eliminated through the bile or urine. It also helps metabolize hormones, regulate blood sugar, and support immune function. When liver pathways become overburdened, toxins may circulate longer, contributing to fatigue or imbalance.

Kidneys – The Filtration Pair

Your kidneys filter the blood, removing excess fluid, salts, and waste products through the urine. This system plays a key role in maintaining internal balance, what we call homeostasis. Healthy kidneys help regulate electrolyte levels, blood pressure, and hydration, and serve as a primary exit route for water-soluble toxins.

Colon – The Final Elimination Channel

After nutrients are absorbed in the small intestine, the colon processes the remaining waste. A sluggish or imbalanced colon can slow detoxification, allowing waste and toxins to linger longer than they should. Healthy bowel movements are a critical part of the body's natural elimination cycle.

Lymphatic System – The Body's Drainage Network

Often overlooked, the lymphatic system acts as a circulatory cleanup crew. It transports cellular waste, proteins, and immune cells throughout the body, draining them into the bloodstream for processing and elimination. When the lymph system is stagnant, due to inactivity, dehydration, or overload, detox can slow down and inflammation may build up.

Lungs – Your Built-In Air Filter

The lungs not only supply oxygen but also expel carbon dioxide and airborne irritants. Through the breath, the body eliminates gaseous waste and responds to airborne toxins or pathogens. Shallow breathing or indoor air pollution can compromise this natural cleansing function.

Skin – The Largest Detox Organ

Your skin acts as a barrier and an excretion route. Sweat helps remove certain toxins, especially heavy metals and chemicals. When detox organs are overloaded, the skin may take on more of the burden, which can show up as irritation, rashes, or other signs of imbalance.

Gut Flora – The Microbial Guardians

The trillions of microbes in your gut play an unsung but critical role in detoxification. Beneficial bacteria help break down toxins, neutralize harmful compounds, and maintain a healthy intestinal lining that prevents unwanted substances from re-entering the bloodstream. An imbalanced microbiome can impair detox function and increase the toxic load your body has to manage.

Together, these systems create a multi-layered, highly coordinated process that's constantly at work behind the scenes. Detoxification isn't about a single organ, it's about a network working in harmony. This book is designed to help you understand and support each of these systems more effectively, one step at a time.

Detoxification Protocols: A Targeted Approach

Each detox pathway in the body plays a distinct role in maintaining internal balance. When these pathways become overwhelmed, the effects can ripple through multiple systems, contributing to a wide range of health concerns.

Liver Detox

The liver serves as the body's primary detoxification organ. It works continuously to process and neutralize toxins so they can be safely eliminated. When the liver becomes congested or overburdened, toxins may recirculate through the bloodstream. This can contribute to systemic inflammation, hormonal fluctuations, and impaired metabolic function. Supporting liver health with targeted nutrients and herbal compounds may help the liver perform more efficiently and reduce the toxic load on the body.

Colon Detox

The colon is central to waste elimination. When digestion slows, toxins and waste may begin to accumulate, resulting in symptoms such as constipation, bloating, gas, and reabsorption of harmful substances. A sluggish colon can also create an environment that encourages the overgrowth of unwanted microbes. Using fiber, probiotics, and herbal support to promote regular bowel movements can help restore healthy digestion and assist in the elimination of accumulated waste.

Parasite Detox

Parasites are more common than many people realize. Intestinal parasites, tapeworms, and microscopic protozoa can disrupt digestion, interfere with nutrient absorption, and place a burden on the immune system. Individuals may experience ongoing bloating, fatigue, sugar cravings, or skin irritation without knowing the cause. A parasite-focused protocol may assist in clearing these organisms and rebalancing the gut environment, offering a pathway toward improved vitality and immune resilience.

Heavy Metal Detox

Toxic heavy metals such as mercury, lead, aluminum, and arsenic can accumulate in key organs including the brain, liver, kidneys, and bones. These substances are often introduced through tap water, cookware, environmental pollutants, and certain medications or dental materials. Over time, their buildup may affect neurological health, hormone balance, and immune function. Gentle detox strategies using compounds like zeolite, chlorella, and cilantro are often used to help bind and remove these substances from the body.

Lymphatic Detox

The lymphatic system is the body's internal drainage and defense network. It circulates lymph fluid, clears cellular waste, and supports immune activity. When lymph flow becomes stagnant, symptoms such as swelling, sluggish circulation, chronic fatigue, or general inflammation may arise. Lymphatic detoxification practices such as regular movement, hydration, dry brushing, and herbal teas can help re-activate this important system and support overall detox efficiency.

Kidney Detox

The kidneys play a vital role in filtering blood, removing waste products, and maintaining proper fluid and mineral balance. Dehydration, excess sodium intake, or heavy metal exposure can place strain on these organs, potentially affecting their ability to filter effectively. Supporting the kidneys through hydration and herbal supplements such as nettle leaf, dandelion root, and cranberry extract may help promote urinary flow and assist in clearing accumulated waste from the body.

Candida and Yeast Detox

An overgrowth of Candida or other yeast species in the digestive tract can disrupt the microbial balance and contribute to a range of symptoms, including sugar cravings, digestive discomfort, brain fog, fatigue, and skin imbalances. This type of imbalance is often triggered by high sugar intake, antibiotic use, or chronic stress. A yeast detox typically includes antifungal herbs, dietary adjustments, and targeted probiotics to support the restoration of a healthy gut ecosystem and reduce the likelihood of recurrence.

Why Detoxification Is Important

In past generations, detoxification may not have been as essential. People lived with fewer chemicals in their environment, consumed whole, unprocessed foods, and were not constantly exposed to synthetic substances. Today, that has changed. Toxins are now found in nearly every aspect of modern life, pesticides in food, heavy metals in water, plastics in packaging, artificial ingredients in processed meals, and hormone-disrupting chemicals in common household products.

These substances can interfere with many key systems in the body. Over time, they may contribute to imbalances in hormone levels, metabolic function, immune activity, and neurological clarity. As the toxic burden increases, the body's natural ability to eliminate waste can become overwhelmed. Detoxification is no longer an optional wellness trend. It has become a practical and necessary strategy for protecting long-term health in a world where exposure is often unavoidable.

The goal is not just to "detox" for a few weeks and return to old habits. Instead, this book encourages the adoption of sustainable detox support, gentle, ongoing practices that keep your systems functioning optimally. By regularly supporting liver function, improving digestion, addressing potential parasite exposure, and minimizing heavy metal accumulation, you give your body the tools it needs to stay resilient.

Your Detox Support Roadmap

This book is your trusted guide to safe, natural, and science-informed detoxification. If you're experiencing persistent fatigue, brain fog, stubborn weight gain, frequent infections, skin irritation, digestive discomfort, or ongoing inflammation, your body may be signaling a toxic overload. The encouraging news is that detoxification, when done correctly, can help your body regain balance and restore vitality from within.

You'll discover how to support your liver, the body's central detoxification hub, so it can process and eliminate unwanted compounds more efficiently. You'll also explore the critical importance of colon health. More than just a digestive issue, colon cleansing can enhance energy, immune function, and overall well-being.

We will take a closer look at often-overlooked systems like the lymphatic network. This internal drainage system helps clear waste and immune debris, but when it becomes stagnant, toxins may accumulate and contribute to fatigue, puffiness, or inflammation. You'll learn simple strategies to keep this system flowing through movement, hydration, and nutritional support.

You'll also learn how to assist your kidneys in filtering water-soluble toxins and maintaining proper fluid balance. Supporting kidney function can lead to improved clarity, energy, and resilience.

Many people are surprised to discover that parasite overgrowth may be contributing to symptoms such as bloating, irritability, nutrient deficiencies, and skin imbalances. This book will show you how to recognize common patterns and support the body in clearing potential invaders naturally.

We will also explore the modern challenge of heavy metal accumulation. These substances can build up over time and are increasingly associated with issues like brain fog, low mood, and immune dysregulation. Fortunately, natural compounds may help gently remove these metals when used with care.

Finally, you'll learn about Candida and yeast overgrowth, a common and under-recognized cause of digestive upset, skin issues, fatigue, and sugar cravings. Rebalancing the gut microbiome through nutrition, probiotics, and herbal support can help restore digestive and cognitive harmony.

Throughout this journey, you will be guided by practical insights and approaches that reflect both current science and real-world experiences. While detoxification is not a cure-all, it is a powerful tool that gives your body the opportunity to recalibrate and renew.

Detoxification is not about punishment or deprivation. It is about supporting your natural systems of renewal so you can feel better, think more clearly, and live with greater energy and purpose. Whether you are looking for a gentle seasonal reset or a more structured full-body cleanse, the roadmap ahead will equip you with the tools and knowledge to begin your journey toward a cleaner, stronger, and more balanced you.

What to Expect in This Book

This book offers a practical, research-informed exploration of key detoxification protocols, designed to support the body's natural ability to cleanse and rebalance itself. Each protocol is introduced through a structured lens that blends scientific understanding with real-world user experience. The aim is to provide clear, usable guidance that helps you make informed decisions about incorporating detox strategies into your wellness routine.

Here's what you can expect in each protocol's section:

Science-Informed Solution Benefits

Each detox area, such as liver support, colon cleansing, parasite protocols, or heavy metal detox, is introduced with an overview of its biological role in the body and the mechanisms through which it may contribute to improved internal balance. These insights are grounded in research, observational data, and the known functions of nutrients, herbs, and compounds commonly used to support detoxification. The emphasis is on potential support functions, not treatment or disease outcomes.

Customer-Reported Solution Benefits

To better understand how these detox strategies are experienced in modern life, each section includes an analysis of real-world user reviews. This part of the book highlights:

Use Case Patterns Observed: A summary of the most common reasons people choose each detox protocol, based on recurring patterns found in customer feedback. These include motivations such as addressing fatigue, improving digestion, boosting clarity, or restoring balance.

Feedback Insights: A narrative summary of how users describe their experiences. This includes both practical outcomes (such as better bowel regularity or more energy) and the emotional tone of their feedback (such as feeling lighter, clearer, or more in control). This section captures the lived experience behind the protocol's use.

Most Reported Benefits from Review Analysis: A data-informed summary of the top benefits most frequently mentioned by users. Based on a breakdown of thousands of customer reviews, this section offers a percentage-based snapshot of which effects are most commonly reported in everyday use.

This combined approach helps present each protocol in a grounded, relatable, and informative way, blending biological understanding with practical experience.

Reference Guide to Everyday Health Goals

At the end of this book, you'll find a convenient reference section that connects commonly reported health concerns, such as fatigue, poor digestion, sluggish skin, or immune imbalances, with the detox protocols most frequently mentioned in association with those issues. This guide reflects a synthesis of both scientific reasoning and user feedback and is intended as an educational resource, not a replacement for individualized health care.

By blending structured scientific insights with real-world perspectives, this book aims to give you a balanced, empowering view of how detoxification may fit into your wellness journey, naturally, gently, and effectively.

Liver Detox

Revitalizing the Body's Primary Detoxification Organ

The liver is widely recognized as one of the most important detoxification organs in the body. It plays a central role in filtering the blood, metabolizing nutrients, processing hormones, and supporting hundreds of biochemical processes essential to daily function. Every day, the liver works to break down and neutralize substances absorbed from the environment, through food, air, water, and topical products, and prepares them for safe elimination.

In today's world, the liver often faces an increased burden. Exposure to processed foods, synthetic chemicals, medications, and environmental pollutants can overwhelm its capacity. When the liver becomes strained, its ability to filter toxins efficiently may be reduced, which can influence energy, digestion, metabolism, immune balance, and even skin clarity. People often describe feeling fatigued, foggy, bloated, or hormonally imbalanced when their liver is under stress.

Fortunately, there are practical and natural ways to support liver function. By providing nutrients and lifestyle habits that assist the liver's natural detoxification processes, many people report improvements in how they feel, function, and recover from daily stressors. Below is an overview of how liver detoxification support may contribute to whole-body vitality.

Science-Informed Liver Detox Benefits

Enhances Liver Function and Detoxification Efficiency

The liver neutralizes and transforms toxins into water-soluble compounds so they can be safely excreted through urine or bile. This process involves two major steps, phase 1 and phase 2 detoxification, which rely on specialized enzymes to modify and bind toxins. However, high exposure to alcohol, medications, environmental chemicals, and poor-quality foods can slow these processes. Supporting the liver with essential nutrients and compounds may help maintain enzymatic activity and improve the body's ability to handle toxic load.

Supports Energy Metabolism and Reduces Fatigue

The liver is central to energy metabolism. It helps regulate blood sugar, stores glycogen, and breaks down fats, proteins, and carbohydrates for use as fuel. When liver function is impaired or overloaded, the conversion of nutrients into usable energy may be compromised. This can contribute to symptoms such as persistent fatigue, sluggishness, or brain fog. Providing supportive nutrients may help the liver better manage these metabolic processes, allowing for steadier energy production at the cellular level.

Encourages Hormonal Balance and Clearance

The liver plays a key role in breaking down and eliminating excess hormones, including estrogen and cortisol. When liver detoxification pathways are functioning well, these hormones are processed and cleared from the body in a timely manner. If the liver is burdened, hormonal buildup can occur, potentially contributing to bloating, irritability, skin changes, or menstrual discomfort. Nutritional and botanical support for liver detoxification may aid in restoring hormonal equilibrium by enhancing clearance mechanisms.

Promotes Digestive Health and Nutrient Absorption

Bile is a fluid produced by the liver that is essential for digesting fats and absorbing fat-soluble vitamins such as A, D, E, and K. If liver function is compromised, bile production and flow may decline, which can result in bloating, indigestion, and reduced nutrient uptake. Supporting liver health helps encourage bile flow, which contributes to more comfortable digestion and improved absorption of critical nutrients from food.

Aids in Fat Metabolism and Weight Regulation

The liver is directly involved in processing dietary fats, regulating cholesterol levels, and managing blood sugar stability. When liver detoxification pathways are compromised, fat metabolism may slow, contributing to weight fluctuations and challenges in maintaining metabolic balance. Supporting liver function can promote more efficient fat processing, which may help improve metabolic outcomes and support healthy weight management efforts.

Assists in Regulating Inflammatory Responses and Immune Function

Toxin accumulation and poor detoxification may contribute to systemic inflammation, which can affect how the immune system responds to internal and external stressors. The liver helps clear inflammatory byproducts and plays a role in immune surveillance. When supported properly, the liver contributes to a more balanced immune response and helps reduce the buildup of pro-inflammatory compounds, allowing for improved resilience.

Maintains Healthy Liver Enzyme Activity

Liver enzymes such as ALT (alanine aminotransferase) and AST (aspartate aminotransferase) are commonly used to assess liver function. While occasional elevations can occur from various causes, long-term elevation may indicate that the liver is under stress. Some studies suggest that targeted nutritional support may help maintain healthy enzyme levels and reduce markers of liver strain, although individual results can vary.

Liver Detox Protocol

Targeted Support for Liver Function and Detoxification

Supporting your liver's natural detoxification process involves using key nutrients, herbs, and supportive compounds that strengthen its ability to filter, process, and eliminate toxins. A well-supported liver detox does not require extreme fasting or restrictive dieting. Instead, it focuses on giving the liver the tools it needs to function efficiently and repair itself when under stress.

While many natural compounds can contribute to liver detoxification, several have gained widespread recognition for their supportive roles. These include Milk Thistle, Dandelion Root, Turmeric, N-Acetyl Cysteine (NAC), and Glutathione. Together, these ingredients help protect liver cells, stimulate bile flow, and reinforce antioxidant defenses, allowing the liver to handle everyday exposure to toxins more effectively.

In addition, many proprietary blends available on the market combine these core ingredients with other liver-supportive herbs and nutrients, offering a comprehensive approach to detoxification. Some of these formulations have been associated with improved liver enzyme profiles, reduced feelings of congestion, and enhanced digestive comfort when used consistently and as directed.

Milk Thistle: A Researched Botanical for Liver Protection

Milk thistle is one of the most studied and widely used herbs for supporting liver health. Its active compound, silymarin, is known for its ability to help protect liver cells from oxidative stress and support the regeneration of damaged tissue. Research has shown that silymarin may help promote healthy enzyme levels and enhance the liver's detoxification capacity. It is commonly included in liver health protocols due to its well-documented antioxidant and hepatoprotective properties.

For more information on milk thistle and its broader applications, refer to the *Herbal Therapy* book in this series.

Dandelion Root: Supporting Bile Flow and Digestive Balance

Dandelion root has been traditionally used to support liver and digestive health. It is believed to stimulate bile production, which is essential for breaking down fats and eliminating fat-soluble toxins from the body. In addition to promoting bile flow, dandelion acts as a mild diuretic, which may help reduce fluid retention and support the body's elimination pathways. It is often used as part of gentle liver and digestive cleansing routines.

Turmeric: Botanical Support for Inflammation and Detox Enzyme Activity

Turmeric is well known for its anti-inflammatory and antioxidant properties, primarily due to its active component, curcumin. In the context of liver health, curcumin has been shown to help modulate liver enzyme activity and support detoxification pathways. It also helps reduce oxidative stress and may protect liver cells from environmental toxins. Turmeric's effectiveness is significantly enhanced when taken with black pepper extract (piperine), which improves absorption. This botanical is commonly included in liver support formulations due to its dual role in inflammation management and detox pathway regulation.

For a full review of turmeric's broader therapeutic roles, see the *Herbal Therapy* book.

N-Acetyl Cysteine (NAC): A Precursor to Glutathione Production

NAC is a powerful amino acid compound that plays a vital role in supporting the liver's antioxidant defense system. It serves as a precursor to glutathione, a compound that is essential for neutralizing free radicals and detoxifying reactive substances in the liver. NAC helps support the liver's ability to process alcohol, pharmaceutical byproducts, and environmental toxins. It has been studied for its potential to promote healthy levels of liver enzymes such as ALT and AST, especially in individuals with toxin burden or metabolic stress.

To explore NAC's broader applications, including its role in respiratory health and antioxidant protection, refer to the *Amino Acid Therapy* book.

Glutathione: The Body's Master Antioxidant for Liver Protection

Glutathione is often referred to as the body's master antioxidant and is critical to liver detoxification. It is directly involved in phase 2 detoxification, where it binds to harmful compounds to facilitate their elimination. When glutathione levels are depleted due to stress, illness, or toxin exposure, the liver's ability to neutralize toxins can decline. Supporting glutathione through direct supplementation or by providing its precursors such as NAC may help improve antioxidant capacity and protect liver cells from oxidative damage. Some liver health products include reduced glutathione or liposomal formulations for enhanced absorption and cellular delivery. To further explore Glutathione, refer to the *Amino Acid Therapy* book.

Liver Detox Support Beyond Individual Herbs

Many liver detox products combine several of the ingredients listed above into synergistic formulations. These often include additional herbs such as artichoke, schisandra, burdock root, and yellow dock, as well as compounds that assist with bile production and digestive support. These blends are formulated to offer comprehensive liver support while promoting the elimination of waste through both the digestive and urinary systems.

Since each formulation varies in potency and design, it is best to follow the product-specific recommendations provided on the label. These protocols are usually tailored to the ingredients included and may offer suggested dosages and timelines for optimal use. Users are encouraged to choose high-quality products from reputable sources and consult a qualified health practitioner for personalized guidance when needed.

Customer-Reported Liver Detox Benefits

For many users, liver detox supplements are not just about cleansing. They are about renewal, an opportunity to feel clearer, lighter, and more in control of their health. With an impressive average rating of 4.6 out of 5 and thousands of positive reviews, liver detox supplements have gained the trust of people from all walks of life, including those managing energy challenges, digestive discomfort, stubborn skin issues, weight fluctuations, or elevated lab values.

What stands out across the reviews is how often users describe their experience as unexpectedly powerful. They are not just hoping to "clean out the liver," but to get their health back on track, often after years of trying diets, medications, or lifestyle changes with limited results. Some come looking for support with alcohol metabolism or medication side effects. Others are navigating fatigue, bloating, hormonal transitions, or unexplained symptoms like acne or inflammation. Many are surprised by how much better they feel after just a few weeks, often using phrases like "life-changing," "I feel like myself again," or "this has become part of my daily routine."

This isn't about magic pills. It's about real people noticing real shifts, in energy, digestion, mood, clarity, and lab markers, when their liver is finally given the support it needs.

Use Case Patterns Observed

Liver detox supplements are most often discovered during periods of imbalance, when fatigue lingers, digestion slows, or the body feels bloated, heavy, or off-center. A common trigger is a lab report showing elevated liver enzymes or suspected fatty liver. Others begin after recognizing symptoms they never associated with liver stress: stubborn weight gain, chronic skin breakouts, lingering brain fog, or irregular bowel movements.

Several reviewers mention that they turned to liver detox products after conventional options failed to provide relief. Some had tried restrictive diets, exercise plans, or acne regimens without results. Others were managing hormone changes during menopause, post-surgery recovery, or the aftermath of medications and alcohol. Many were referred by friends, doctors, or even veterinarians who had seen results firsthand.

The motivation is often deeply personal. Whether it is about preventing future problems, avoiding invasive tests, or feeling more at ease in their body, people start this journey to take back control, and frequently find that a gentle, herbal-based supplement offers far more support than expected.

Feedback Insights

Across hundreds of reviews, the emotional tone is one of relief, discovery, and renewed optimism. Users speak of feeling "lighter," "less bloated," and "more energized" within days of starting. One reviewer who struggled for years with weight gain despite clean eating wrote, "I think there's a skinny girl under all this fluid," after seeing her ankles shrink and her pants finally fit loosely. Another, dealing with persistent brain fog and fatigue, reported waking up feeling more rested and alert, with "a peaceful calm" that had been missing for years.

People with previously elevated enzyme levels share powerful testimonials about seeing their lab markers return to normal. These stories are often told with a sense of cautious excitement, grateful to see progress and hoping it continues. "The proof is in my labs," one wrote after her AST and ALT dropped into the normal range without changing her habits. Others echoed, saying things like, "This gave me peace of mind," or "Finally, something that works."

Skin transformations are also a recurring theme. Some users who battled stubborn acne or eczema for years describe clearer skin after just one bottle, often calling it "the missing piece" in their health routine. "I forgot what my face looked like before," wrote one user, while another said, "I'm aging backwards."

Sleep is another surprising area of improvement. A few reviewers managing chronic insomnia or post-surgery fatigue noticed deeper rest and calmer nights.

Many reviewers reflect on how liver detox support has become a permanent part of their daily rhythm. Some take it with orange juice, others prefer it in capsule form, but the sentiment is the same: it fits into their life, it helps them feel better, and they are not looking back.

As one person summarized simply, "It doesn't just help your liver. It helps you feel like you again."

Most Reported Benefits from Review Analysis

To better understand how liver detox supplements are experienced in real-world use, we conducted an in-depth analysis of verified customer reviews. These insights reflect the benefits most frequently mentioned by satisfied users. While everyone's experience is unique, the percentages below reveal patterns that may help you decide whether liver detox support is right for your needs.

For example, 58% of users specifically mentioned noticeable improvements in liver health. Many described feeling less bloated, more energized, and better able to handle daily life after incorporating liver detox supplements into their routine. Similar trends appeared in digestion, toxin removal, and energy levels, giving a clear view of what users appreciate most.

Below is a summary table of liver detox's top benefits as reported by customers:

Benefit	%	Explanation
Liver Health	58%	Most users report feeling improvements in liver function, less bloating, and better detox balance.
Digestion & Gut Health	13%	Many mention smoother digestion, less stomach discomfort, and greater digestive regularity.
Toxin Removal	13%	Users often describe a sense of "clearing out," with fewer symptoms of toxic buildup or heaviness.
Energy Boost	11%	A number of reviewers report greater stamina, sharper focus, and reduced fatigue throughout the day.
Skin Health	5%	Some users notice clearer skin, fewer breakouts, and a healthier complexion over time.

How to Use This Table

If you are exploring liver detox support for a particular reason, whether it is to feel more energized, reduce bloating, or maintain healthy liver function, this table can serve as a helpful reference point. The percentages reflect how often each benefit was mentioned among users who had a positive experience. They are not guarantees, but they do highlight what results are most commonly noticed.

Many reviewers report multiple improvements at once, especially when the supplement is used consistently over several weeks. Whether you are managing lifestyle-related stress, aiming to improve digestion, or simply looking to feel more balanced, these insights offer a useful snapshot of how liver detox support may fit into your wellness plan.

Colon Detox

Restoring Gut Health for Optimal Digestion and Detoxification

The colon is one of the body's essential elimination pathways, responsible for processing waste, absorbing remaining nutrients, and facilitating the final stage of detoxification. It works closely with the liver and the rest of the digestive system to ensure that toxins and metabolic waste are efficiently excreted. However, modern habits, including low fiber intake, processed foods, inadequate hydration, stress, and environmental toxin exposure, can disrupt colon function, leading to sluggish elimination, waste buildup, and digestive discomfort.

When the colon is not functioning optimally, toxins that should be removed from the body can linger in the digestive tract. This can contribute to constipation, bloating, fatigue, weakened immune response, brain fog, and systemic inflammation. Over time, poor colon health may also lead to reduced nutrient absorption, imbalances in gut flora, and a greater toxic load on the body. A sluggish colon affects far more than digestion, it may also influence metabolism, skin health, hormonal balance, and overall well-being.

Supporting colon detoxification is one way to restore digestive efficiency, improve elimination, and promote a healthy internal environment. With the right combination of hydration, fiber, dietary support, and targeted supplementation, the colon can function more effectively, helping to reduce toxic burden and support overall health.

Science-Informed Colon Detox Benefits

Promotes Regular Bowel Movements and Prevents Constipation

A well-functioning colon is essential for the healthy elimination of waste. When the colon becomes sluggish, often due to insufficient fiber, dehydration, or poor eating habits, waste can accumulate, leading to constipation, abdominal discomfort, and bloating. Colon detoxification encourages regularity by stimulating peristalsis, the rhythmic muscle contractions that move waste through the intestines. It also helps clear built-up material, allowing the colon to resume normal movement and reduce discomfort associated with irregular elimination.

Enhances Nutrient Absorption and Digestive Efficiency

When the colon is burdened by accumulated waste or slowed motility, it may interfere with the final stages of digestion and nutrient absorption. This can prevent the body from effectively utilizing key vitamins, minerals, and electrolytes. By cleansing the colon and reducing the presence of residual waste, detoxification helps restore optimal surface contact between food and intestinal lining, allowing for better absorption and greater digestive efficiency.

Reduces Bloating and Gas

Undigested food and slow-moving material in the colon can ferment, leading to excess gas and bloating. These symptoms are often compounded by microbial imbalances, where harmful bacteria outnumber beneficial species. Colon detoxification helps reduce fermentation by clearing stagnant matter and supporting the rebalancing of gut flora. Many users report feeling less distended and more comfortable after beginning a colon detox routine.

Supports the Gut Microbiome and Reduces Harmful Bacteria

The colon is home to trillions of microbes that help regulate immunity, produce key nutrients, and aid digestion. However, when the colon becomes congested, or when diet and stress compromise microbial diversity, harmful organisms such as yeast and pathogenic bacteria can take hold. Colon detoxification helps flush out these disruptive microbes, making space for beneficial bacteria to thrive. A balanced microbiome is essential for maintaining gut integrity and overall resilience.

Aids in Weight Management and Reduces Toxin Storage

The body often stores toxins in fat tissue as a protective mechanism when elimination pathways are overburdened. Over time, this can contribute to weight gain or metabolic resistance. Colon detoxification may help support weight regulation by clearing waste, reducing inflammation, and encouraging proper digestion and nutrient use. While not a weight loss solution on its own, colon detox can help restore conditions that support healthy metabolic function and more efficient fat processing.

Reduces Inflammation and Supports Immune Function

A congested colon may lead to reabsorption of toxic substances into the bloodstream, which can trigger systemic inflammation. Chronic exposure to these circulating toxins may compromise the immune system and contribute to low-grade inflammatory responses. Detoxifying the colon can reduce this burden, helping to calm inflammatory pathways and support immune regulation. A well-functioning colon allows the body to eliminate irritants efficiently and maintain clearer immune communication.

Helps Prevent Colon-Related Disorders

Maintaining a clean and functional colon may help lower the risk of common digestive conditions such as diverticulitis, irritable bowel syndrome (IBS), and chronic constipation. Colon detoxification supports overall intestinal tone, improves motility, and can reduce the buildup of matter that contributes to irritation or inflammation. Long-term, this may help preserve the structural and functional integrity of the gut lining and reduce strain on the digestive system.

Colon Detox Protocol

Colon Detox Protocol

A healthy colon plays a foundational role in the body's overall detoxification and digestive processes. It is responsible not only for eliminating waste, but also for absorbing water, reclaiming essential nutrients, and maintaining the balance of beneficial gut bacteria. When the colon becomes sluggish or congested due to poor diet, dehydration, stress, medications, or environmental toxins, waste may linger in the digestive tract, leading to symptoms such as bloating, irregular bowel movements, discomfort, and fatigue. Over time, this accumulation can impact nutrient absorption, gut microbiome balance, and systemic inflammation.

Supporting colon detoxification can help the body return to a more efficient, balanced state. A well-designed colon detox protocol promotes regularity, helps clear out built-up waste, and improves gut function without relying on harsh or aggressive methods. The most effective approaches focus on gentle, fiber-rich, herbal, and probiotic-based support, allowing the body to cleanse itself naturally and safely.

Psyllium Husk: The Fiber-Powered Cleanser

Psyllium husk is one of the most widely used and research-supported fibers for digestive health. As a soluble fiber, it absorbs water in the intestines and forms a gel-like substance that increases stool bulk and moisture. This makes elimination easier and more regular while also helping sweep away waste material that may have accumulated along the colon wall. Psyllium also serves as a prebiotic, nourishing beneficial gut bacteria and supporting a healthy microbiome. Unlike stimulant laxatives, psyllium supports regular bowel movements through mechanical action, making it a safe, long-term solution for improved digestion.

For a more in-depth discussion of fiber's role in detoxification and wellness, see the *HOPED Protocol* book in this series.

Aloe Vera: Soothing, Hydrating, and Gut-Calming

Aloe vera has been used for centuries as a natural aid for digestive discomfort. In the context of colon detox, aloe offers gentle laxative effects while also calming irritation in the intestinal lining. It may be particularly helpful for individuals dealing with occasional constipation, irritable bowel symptoms, or bloating. Unlike stronger laxatives, aloe supports smoother transit while helping maintain hydration and reducing internal inflammation. Its gentle nature makes it a favored ingredient in many modern detox blends.

Senna Leaf: Short-Term Stimulant for Deep Elimination

Senna leaf is a powerful herbal laxative commonly used to relieve temporary constipation or to jumpstart the detoxification process. It works by stimulating the colon's muscular contractions, known as peristalsis, which help move waste through the digestive tract more quickly. While highly effective for short-term use, senna is best reserved for brief periods due to its potential to create dependency if overused. When used occasionally and in the right dose, it can assist in clearing out accumulated waste and kickstarting the detox process.

Bentonite Clay and Activated Charcoal: Toxin Binders

Some colon detox products include natural binders like **bentonite clay** or **activated charcoal**, which help trap toxins, gas, and heavy metals in the digestive tract. These compounds are not absorbed by the body, but instead carry bound toxins out through the stool. While not essential for every detox, they are popular in deeper cleansing protocols and may be helpful for individuals with a higher toxic burden or those undergoing a more intensive reset.

Probiotics: Restoring Balance After Detox

Once waste is cleared from the colon, it is important to re-establish a healthy gut flora. Probiotics help repopulate the gut with beneficial bacteria, support immune function, and promote long-term digestive resilience. Many colon detox protocols include a probiotic phase after the initial cleanse to ensure microbial balance is restored and maintained. This is especially important when the detox involves temporary disruption to the gut ecosystem.

Choosing the Right Approach

Most colon detox supplements combine several of the ingredients listed above to provide a more complete and balanced effect. These multi-phase formulas may begin with fiber and gentle laxatives, followed by binding agents and probiotic reintroduction. Others offer slow-release daily detox support that can be taken over longer periods without disrupting daily life.

Because formulations vary in strength and purpose, it is important to follow the dosing guidelines provided on the product label. Some programs are designed for short-term cleansing, while others support ongoing digestive maintenance. Those with sensitive systems or pre-existing conditions should consult a qualified healthcare practitioner before starting any new detox protocol.

Customer-Reported Colon Detox Benefits

Colon detox supplements receive strong praise from users seeking relief from chronic bloating, sluggish digestion, and a desire for a deep internal reset. With an overall rating of 4.3 out of 5 stars, this category of products resonates with those who feel weighed down physically and emotionally by digestive sluggishness. Many describe feeling lighter, more energetic, and surprisingly refreshed, both physically and mentally, after even a few days of consistent use.

The tone of these reviews reflects not just functional changes in digestion, but also a profound emotional release. For many, it was a mix of comic relief, disbelief, and gratitude. Users often joked about "finding God in the bathroom," “hearing hymns,” or “repenting for dietary sins,” suggesting that while the experience could be intense, it was also deeply cathartic. That said, users repeatedly emphasized the importance of preparation, hydration, and starting slowly.

This section draws on patterns from thousands of verified 4- and 5-star reviews to illustrate how people are actually using colon detox supplements, and how they feel about their results.

Use Case Patterns Observed

Many people turn to colon detox supplements when they feel heavy, bloated, or irregular, especially after periods of overeating, processed food, or travel. These users often mention wanting a fresh start or a digestive "reset," typically following holidays, vacations, or lifestyle changes.

Some were dealing with long-term constipation or sluggish bowel movements and had already tried gentle laxatives or fiber supplements with little success. Others described themselves as regular supplement users who cleanse every few months as part of a maintenance routine. In many cases, people were not just aiming to go to the bathroom, they wanted to reduce bloating, support their metabolism, manage cravings, improve energy, or kick-start a healthier diet.

The most common starting approach was to take at night and wait for results the next morning. Many users found this to be surprisingly effective, though some quickly moved to heavier dose for a deeper cleanse, often with comically intense outcomes. For most, the first few days produced the most dramatic results, followed by a more manageable pace as the days progressed.

Feedback Insights

The emotional tone of customer reviews was a mix of awe, relief, discomfort, and humor. While many described the experience as "not for the faint of heart," the overwhelming response was that it worked, and worked powerfully. One reviewer wrote, "It didn't just clean me out, it cleaned my soul." Another confessed to "repenting for everything I ever ate" while reflecting on life choices during their bathroom visits.

People consistently described an intense initial phase, marked by strong cramping, urgent trips to the restroom, and unexpectedly fast results. The phrase "do not trust a fart" appeared in various forms across reviews, often paired with warnings to stay home and stock up on toilet paper. Despite the discomfort, users often expressed deep satisfaction with the outcome, noting they felt lighter, had flatter stomachs, and experienced better sleep and mental clarity.

Several users expressed joy at finally having relief from years of constipation, with one calling it "the first real bowel movement in over a decade." Another described smiling at her reflection after "finally pooping for real" and feeling a sense of freedom she hadn't had in years. For others, it was about control, resetting cravings, managing bloating, and feeling a renewed connection to their body.

Even when side effects like mild nausea, bloating, or cramping were mentioned, users frequently framed them as worth the end result. Many commented that while the journey was intense, the clarity, lightness, and improved digestion made it something they would repeat again.

Most Reported Benefits from Review Analysis

To better understand how colon detox supplements are experienced in the real world, we analyzed thousands of verified 4- and 5-star customer reviews. The table below reflects the most frequently reported benefits among users with positive outcomes. While individual results vary, a higher percentage indicates a more consistent pattern of benefit across a large group of users.

For example, 27 percent of reviewers mentioned noticeable improvements in toxin elimination, suggesting that many users felt cleaner, lighter, and more refreshed after using colon detox products. Bloating relief and digestive regularity were also among the top experiences shared, indicating strong relevance for anyone struggling with gut sluggishness or irregularity.

Colon Detox's Top Benefits Reported by Customers

Benefit	%	Explanation
Toxin Removal	27%	Many users report improved detoxification, cleansing of the digestive tract, and a lighter feeling overall.
Bloating and Gas Relief	25%	Helps reduce bloating, gas, and digestive discomfort, making the stomach feel flatter and more at ease.
Digestive Regularity	24%	Supports regular bowel movements and helps relieve occasional constipation, which improves overall gut function.
Weight Management	21%	Some users report feeling lighter and experiencing mild weight loss, often due to reduced waste buildup and improved elimination.
Energy Boost	4%	A smaller group of users noted increased energy and mental clarity after detoxifying the colon.

How to Use This Guide

If you are considering colon detox supplements to support digestion, reduce bloating, or feel more energized, this guide offers a clear starting point. The percentages reflect how often each benefit was mentioned among users who shared positive results, rather than guaranteed outcomes.

That said, these patterns highlight what people most commonly experience when using colon detox products. For many, results are noticeable within the first few days, especially when paired with proper hydration and a lighter diet. Some users reported multiple benefits at once, such as better digestion, increased energy, and less bloating.

If you are starting a colon cleanse for the first time, consider beginning with a lower dose and choosing a time when you can remain close to home. As with all supplements, results vary by individual, but these collective insights can help guide your expectations and support a more informed, comfortable detox experience.

Parasite Detox

Targeting Hidden Invaders that Disrupt Health

Your body is a complex biological system that thrives when all of its components are in balance. However, that balance can be silently disrupted by organisms that are rarely discussed in conventional health conversations: parasites. These unwanted invaders, such as pinworms, roundworms, tapeworms, flukes, and microscopic protozoa like Giardia, can enter the body through contaminated water, undercooked food, or exposure to unhygienic environments. Once inside, they often take up residence in the digestive tract, bloodstream, liver, or tissues, where they feed off your nutrients and interfere with your body's ability to function at its best.

Parasites often go undetected because their symptoms mimic other conditions. Digestive discomfort, bloating, persistent fatigue, skin irritation, nutrient deficiencies, and compromised immune function may all be signs of a hidden parasitic burden. For many people, these symptoms persist despite changes in diet or lifestyle, because the underlying issue remains unresolved.

A targeted parasite detox aims to address these hidden invaders by supporting the body's ability to eliminate them and restore balance. This type of detox typically involves the use of herbal compounds and plant-based ingredients known to have antiparasitic activity. Rather than using harsh chemical treatments, natural parasite detox protocols work in harmony with the body, helping to clear out these organisms while also supporting the organs involved in detoxification, including the liver, colon, and lymphatic system.

By committing to a well-structured parasite detox, you support your body's efforts to reclaim essential nutrients, repair the gut lining, rebalance the microbiome, and reduce systemic inflammation. The result is often improved energy, clearer skin, stronger immunity, and enhanced mental clarity. In the sections that follow, we will explore the science-informed benefits of parasite detoxification and the practical role it can play in your long-term health.

Science-Informed Parasite Detox Benefits

Supports Digestive Health and Restores Gut Balance

Parasites can irritate the intestinal lining, compete with beneficial bacteria, and disrupt normal digestion. Many people experience chronic bloating, irregular bowel movements, or food sensitivities that resolve after completing a parasite cleanse. By helping remove the source of irritation, a detox protocol allows the gut to begin healing, making digestion more efficient and comfortable.

Enhances Nutrient Absorption and Prevents Deficiencies

When parasites consume your nutrients, your body can't access the vitamins and minerals it needs, even if your diet is nutritious. Over time, this can lead to deficiencies in iron, vitamin B12, magnesium, and other critical nutrients. Detoxification helps eliminate these nutrient thieves and restores the body's ability to absorb and utilize food more effectively.

Boosts Energy Levels and Reduces Fatigue

A sluggish, parasite-burdened body must work harder to maintain basic functions. This ongoing internal stress often results in persistent fatigue, low motivation, and brain fog. When parasites are removed, many people report feeling a renewed sense of energy, better focus, and mental clarity that had previously been out of reach.

Improves Skin Clarity and Reduces Inflammatory Skin Conditions

Parasites release metabolic waste into the bloodstream that the body must filter and eliminate. When the liver and gut are overwhelmed, the skin becomes a secondary detoxification route, leading to breakouts, rashes, and other inflammatory skin conditions. By addressing the root cause, a parasite detox can support clearer, more radiant skin from within.

Strengthens the Immune System and Reduces Infection Risk

Chronic parasite exposure can confuse or suppress the immune system, leaving the body vulnerable to other infections. Many parasites also produce immunosuppressive chemicals that lower the body's ability to fight back. Detoxification helps clear these hidden stressors so that your immune system can function with greater strength and responsiveness.

Supports Detoxification of Harmful Pathogens and Toxins

Parasites often harbor harmful microbes such as bacteria, viruses, and fungi. Some also release neurotoxins and ammonia-like substances that tax the brain and liver. A proper parasite detox not only removes the organisms themselves but also supports the liver, kidneys, and colon in flushing out the metabolic waste left behind.

Aids in Weight Management and Reduces Food Cravings

Certain parasites can influence hunger signals and blood sugar levels. For example, they may trigger cravings for sugar and refined carbohydrates, which feed both the parasite and cycles of inflammation. Detoxification helps interrupt these feedback loops and can result in reduced cravings, improved satiety, and easier weight control.

Reduces Chronic Inflammation and Alleviates Autoimmune Symptoms

Parasites can provoke a low-grade, chronic inflammatory response that contributes to joint pain, muscle stiffness, and flare-ups of autoimmune conditions. By removing these inflammatory triggers, the body may experience a reduction in immune overactivation, which can provide relief for individuals dealing with conditions like rheumatoid arthritis, lupus, or thyroid imbalance.

Protects Against Long-Term Organ Damage

Some parasites, such as liver flukes or certain protozoa, can migrate and cause damage to organs beyond the digestive tract. The liver, brain, lungs, and even the heart may be affected over time. A proactive parasite cleanse helps eliminate these threats before they can contribute to long-term health consequences.

Parasite Detox Protocol

Parasites are a hidden yet common cause of digestive discomfort, nutrient deficiencies, and chronic health issues. These microscopic invaders can enter the body through contaminated food, water, insect bites, and even unwashed produce. Once inside, they disrupt digestion, deplete essential nutrients, and contribute to bloating, fatigue, and weakened immunity. A parasite detox helps eliminate these unwanted organisms, restoring gut balance and improving overall health.

A successful parasite detox does not rely on harsh chemicals or synthetic treatments but instead focuses on natural, time-tested herbs and compounds that work with the body to expel parasites safely. Some of the most effective natural ingredients for parasite detoxification include Black Walnut, Clove, and Wormwood. These botanicals have been traditionally used to eliminate intestinal parasites, support digestion, and prevent reinfestation. Additionally, multi-herb parasite detox formulas combine these powerful ingredients with other gut-supportive compounds to enhance the cleansing process.

Black Walnut: Disrupting Parasite Life Cycles

Black walnut is one of the most well-known natural antiparasitic remedies, containing compounds that target parasites at various stages of their lifecycle. It helps weaken and expel parasites while supporting overall gut health. Black walnut is particularly effective against intestinal worms and protozoa that disrupt digestion and nutrient absorption.

Clove: Powerful Antimicrobial and Egg Destroyer

Clove contains eugenol, a compound known for its ability to eliminate parasite eggs and prevent re-infestation. Unlike other herbs that target adult parasites, clove helps disrupt the reproductive cycle, ensuring that parasites do not continue to multiply in the body. This makes it a crucial ingredient in any parasite detox strategy.

Wormwood: Natural Vermifuge for Parasite Removal

Wormwood is a potent herbal vermifuge, meaning it expels worms and parasites from the digestive system. It supports the body's ability to eliminate these harmful invaders while soothing inflammation in the gut. Wormwood is particularly useful for addressing roundworms, pinworms, and other common parasites that affect digestive health.

Parasite Detox Support Beyond Individual Herbs

Many parasite detox supplements combine these herbs into a single formula, offering a comprehensive approach to cleansing. These formulations may also include other gut-supporting ingredients like garlic, oregano oil, and berberine, which enhance the detox process by promoting microbial balance in the intestines.

Since different parasite detox formulations vary in strength and duration, it is best to follow product-specific recommendations based on the supplement you choose. Many structured parasite cleanses involve a combination of herbs, digestive enzymes, and probiotics, helping the body eliminate parasites while restoring gut health.

By incorporating targeted parasite-cleansing herbs and compounds into your wellness routine, you support better digestion, improved nutrient absorption, and a stronger immune system, ensuring your body remains resilient against future infections.

Customer-Reported Parasite Detox Benefits

Many people begin a parasite cleanse with uncertainty, unsure if hidden organisms are really affecting their health. But once they try a detox, the results often speak for themselves. Across thousands of reviews, individuals shared how their lives changed after addressing what they believed were long-ignored or misdiagnosed concerns. With an average satisfaction rating of 4.2 out of 5 stars, this solution stands out not just for its ingredients, but for the powerful transformations people report, physically, emotionally, and energetically.

For some, it was the first time in years they felt truly "themselves" again. Others found relief from persistent fatigue, digestive discomfort, and mental fog that no doctor could explain. Many describe a renewed sense of vitality, a calm stomach, and a surprising boost in mental clarity. Whether driven by long-term gut issues, mysterious symptoms, or a simple desire to feel better, the collective voice of customers offers real-world insight into what this approach may offer.

Use Case Patterns Observed

Most people turned to parasite detox after struggling with vague, unresolved symptoms that conventional medicine couldn't pinpoint, chronic bloating, fatigue, irregular digestion, itchy skin, or sinus problems. A large number had been told they had IBS, food intolerances, anxiety, or hormone issues, but nothing seemed to help. Some had been dealing with ongoing infections, mysterious rashes, or constant sugar cravings. Others were recovering from overseas travel, lived with pets, or had frequent exposure to raw or undercooked food.

A recurring pattern was the experience of being dismissed or overlooked by healthcare providers, despite ongoing symptoms. These individuals took matters into their own hands and discovered that cleansing their system produced noticeable, often dramatic results. Many began with skepticism and a strong dose of curiosity, while others, having exhausted all other options, saw it as a last resort.

In many cases, users reported planning repeat rounds or adding liver and colon support as part of a broader detox routine. Some even shared that the detox gave them confidence to address long-standing health concerns and inspired them to make other lifestyle changes. A surprising number also involved family members or partners in the process, often after seeing undeniable results.

Feedback Insights

The emotional impact of the parasite detox journey was significant and deeply personal for many reviewers. Words like "relieved," "grateful," and "amazed" appeared frequently, especially from those who had dealt with symptoms for years without answers. One reviewer described the experience as "life-changing," after regaining their energy, mental clarity, and digestive comfort for the first time in over a decade.

Another user wrote, "I finally have hope. I thought I was crazy for years," echoing a common theme of validation and empowerment. Others described the cleanse as both "gross and glorious," with emotions ranging from initial anxiety to triumphant discovery. Even those who experienced "die-off" symptoms, like headaches, fatigue, or flu-like sensations, often interpreted them as signs that something was working.

Some reviews reflected a deep frustration with the medical system, particularly among those who had been told their lab results were "normal" while they continued to suffer. These individuals often reported a sense of vindication after seeing what they believed were clear signs of parasites exiting their bodies. The connection between improved skin clarity, less joint discomfort, lighter mood, and regular bowel movements came up repeatedly, reinforcing the feeling that a hidden root cause had finally been addressed.

While not everyone had visible results or dramatic reactions, even those with milder experiences often said they felt "lighter," "cleaner," and more energized. And nearly all agreed: this was something worth doing at least once a year.

Most Reported Benefits from Review Analysis

Our analysis focused on reviews where users reported a clear positive experience. From those, we identified the most frequently mentioned benefits. These percentages represent how often a specific outcome was highlighted among satisfied users. While individual experiences may vary, the data offers helpful insight into what others noticed most consistently during their detox journey.

The top benefit, reported by nearly one-third of users, was the visible or felt removal of parasites. Many reviewers described a dramatic shift in their health after this release, including improvements in digestion, energy, skin clarity, and immune resilience. Whether people were addressing persistent digestive discomfort, unexplained fatigue, or recurring skin issues, the sense of "finally figuring it out" came through loud and clear.

Parasite Detox's Top Benefits Reported by Customers

Benefit	%	Explanation
Parasite Removal	31%	Many users report successfully flushing out parasites and experiencing a renewed sense of vitality and internal cleanliness.
Digestive Relief	26%	Users often notice reduced bloating, gas, and stomach discomfort, alongside more regular bowel movements.
Immune Support	19%	Several users describe fewer recurring infections and feeling stronger overall, possibly due to a reduced burden on the immune system.
Energy Boost	13%	A notable number of reviewers felt more alert and less sluggish after the detox, with improved stamina and mental clarity.

Benefit	%	Explanation
Skin Health	11%	Some users experienced a visible reduction in breakouts, skin irritation, and puffiness following parasite elimination.

How to Use This Table

This table is meant to give you a general sense of how people most commonly benefit from parasite detox supplements. The percentages reflect patterns from users who had positive results, and may help you anticipate what to look for in your own experience. For example, if you struggle with digestive issues or fatigue and see those benefits were frequently mentioned, it suggests you might notice similar changes.

While not everyone will have the same results, this data can guide your expectations and encourage you to observe any shifts in how you feel over time. If you decide to try a parasite detox, consider supporting your body with hydration, rest, and a healthy diet to get the most from the process. As always, consult with a healthcare provider if you have underlying conditions or unique concerns.

Heavy Metal Detox

Detox for Brain, Energy, and Metabolic Balance

In today's industrialized world, exposure to heavy metals is nearly impossible to avoid. Toxic elements such as lead, mercury, arsenic, cadmium, and aluminum can enter the body through contaminated water, air pollution, processed foods, dental materials, and even cookware and personal care products. Once inside, these metals tend to accumulate in the body's tissues and organs, where they can interfere with normal physiological functions and contribute to a wide range of health concerns.

Lead is known for its neurotoxic effects and is particularly harmful to children, where it may impact cognitive development and behavior. In adults, it has been associated with high blood pressure and kidney dysfunction. Mercury, often found in fish and amalgam fillings, can disrupt the nervous system, contributing to mood swings, memory issues, and difficulty concentrating. Arsenic exposure, especially through contaminated drinking water, may increase the risk of cardiovascular disease. Cadmium, present in tobacco smoke and industrial environments, can impair kidney function and weaken bones. Aluminum, commonly used in food packaging and some medications, has raised concerns for its potential link to neurodegenerative disorders.

These metals often build up slowly, silently interfering with cellular function. They may impair mitochondrial energy production, disrupt hormone regulation, weaken immune defenses, and provoke chronic inflammation throughout the body. Over time, this toxic burden can result in symptoms such as fatigue, digestive disturbances, poor memory, skin irritation, and more persistent health complaints.

A well-structured heavy metal detox can support the body's ability to eliminate these elements more efficiently. When done correctly, detoxification may help restore internal balance, improve energy levels, and reduce the risk of long-term damage. Let's explore what the science says about how this process works and what benefits you may expect.

Science-Backed Heavy Metal Detoxification Benefits

Helps Protect Brain Health and Cognitive Function

Heavy metals like mercury, lead, and aluminum can cross the blood-brain barrier and accumulate in brain tissue, where they disrupt normal neurological function. These metals have been implicated in memory loss, cognitive fog, and increased risk of neurodegenerative diseases. A heavy metal detox may help reduce this toxic load, supporting clearer thinking, improved mood, and sharper mental performance. Individuals often report better focus and less mental fatigue after supporting brain detoxification.

Supports Energy Production and Reduces Chronic Fatigue

Heavy metals can impair mitochondrial function, the process by which cells produce energy. When energy metabolism is disrupted, the result is often persistent fatigue, sluggishness, and muscle weakness. Detoxifying the body helps restore efficient cellular energy production, leading to noticeable improvements in physical stamina, mental clarity, and resilience during the day.

Enhances Detoxification Pathways in the Liver and Kidneys

The liver and kidneys serve as the body's primary detox organs, but an overload of heavy metals can interfere with their function. Mercury and cadmium in particular can impair enzyme activity in these organs, slowing toxin clearance. A well-designed detox program may help relieve this burden, promoting more effective elimination and improving overall metabolic health.

Promotes Hormonal Balance and Reduces Endocrine Disruption

Some heavy metals mimic or block hormone activity in the body. For example, mercury and lead may interfere with thyroid function, while cadmium and aluminum can disrupt reproductive hormones. This interference may contribute to symptoms such as mood swings, weight gain, low libido, or menstrual irregularities. By reducing the presence of these disruptive elements, detoxification can help restore balance across the endocrine system.

Helps Reduce Chronic Inflammation and Strengthen Immunity

Heavy metals are known to trigger low-grade inflammation that may linger for years. They can also impair the immune system's ability to function properly, making the body more susceptible to infections, allergies, and autoimmune reactions. Detoxing these elements helps calm inflammatory pathways and may allow the immune system to return to more effective function, promoting greater resilience.

Supports Heart and Circulatory Health

Metals like lead and cadmium can damage blood vessels, raise blood pressure, and increase the risk of cardiovascular problems. These metals may also reduce the elasticity of arteries and contribute to oxidative stress within the vascular system. By removing these toxins, circulation often improves and the strain on the cardiovascular system is reduced, which may lead to better heart health over time.

Improves Skin Health and Supports Natural Elimination

When the liver and kidneys are overwhelmed, the body may attempt to eliminate toxins through the skin, leading to acne, eczema, rashes, or dull complexion. Reducing the toxic load through internal detoxification can help relieve this burden, often resulting in a clearer, brighter appearance and improved skin tone.

Helps Prevent Long-Term Organ Damage

The effects of heavy metals are not just short-term. Over time, they may contribute to damage in the kidneys, brain, liver, bones, and nervous system. Mercury and arsenic, for instance, are associated with long-term risks including nerve degeneration. A detox approach that helps mobilize and remove these metals may protect against future health decline.

Reduces the Risk of Chronic Conditions Linked to Heavy Metal Exposure

A growing body of research links heavy metal accumulation to a wide range of chronic conditions, including autoimmune disorders, metabolic syndrome, reproductive challenges, and neurological issues. By lowering your body's heavy metal burden, you may reduce your vulnerability to these types of long-term health challenges and help restore the foundation for more vibrant well-being.

Supports Overall Wellness and Restores Vitality

A heavy metal detox is not just about eliminating toxins; it is about revitalizing the body's systems so they can work the way they are designed to. With fewer internal obstacles, energy flows more smoothly, the immune system responds more appropriately, digestion improves, and mood often lifts. Many people describe a feeling of renewal, both physically and emotionally, after completing a thoughtful detox protocol.

Heavy Metal Detox Protocol

Embarking on a heavy metal detox protocol is a proactive step towards purifying your body and restoring optimal health. This comprehensive approach utilizes specially prepared herbal supplements designed to bind and eliminate toxic heavy metals from your system, supporting your body's natural detoxification processes. By integrating these powerful herbs into your detox routine, you can effectively cleanse your body of harmful metals such as lead, mercury, arsenic, cadmium, and aluminum, thereby enhancing your overall well-being.

Zeolite: A Key Supplement for Heavy Metal Detox

Zeolite, a natural mineral with its potent chelating properties, plays a vital role in heavy metal detoxification. Zeolite works by binding to heavy metals in the body, facilitating their safe removal through the digestive tract, making it a critical tool for reducing the toxic burden on vital organs. Available in both capsule and powder form, it is typically taken in dosages ranging from 1 to 3 grams daily, split into multiple doses to maximize its detoxifying effects. Incorporating Zeolite into your detox protocol helps ensure heavy metals are effectively captured and expelled, preventing further accumulation and supporting overall health.

Zeolite for Developmental Delays in Children

For toddlers and young children, particularly those experiencing slow developmental progress or managing autism, Zeolite is available in a liquid tincture form specially designed for gentle detoxification. Many parents have reported remarkable improvements in their children's behavior, focus, and overall development after incorporating Zeolite tincture into their routine. Its ability to safely bind and eliminate toxins provides vital support for children whose developmental challenges may be linked to heavy metal exposure. As an integral part of a holistic approach to managing autism or developmental delays, Zeolite offers a natural, non-invasive solution to promote healing and better outcomes.

Chlorella

Chlorella, a type of green algae, is another essential component of an effective heavy metal detox. This nutrient-dense supplement excels at binding to heavy metals, aiding in their detoxification and removal from the body. Chlorella is available in tablet or powder form and is commonly taken in doses of 2 to 4 grams daily, divided into multiple servings throughout the day. When combined with Zeolite and other detoxifying agents, chlorella enhances the body's ability to eliminate toxins, ensuring a thorough cleanse that supports overall health and vitality.

Cilantro

Cilantro (Coriandrum sativum) plays a pivotal role in enhancing the body's natural detox pathways. This versatile herb not only adds a fresh flavor to meals but also significantly boosts the elimination of heavy metals through urine and feces. Cilantro can be consumed in various forms, including fresh leaves in meals, concentrated extracts, or as a tea. A typical dosage might include 1 to 2 teaspoons of fresh cilantro leaves per day or 500 mg of concentrated extract taken twice daily. By integrating cilantro into your diet, you support the body's ability to naturally expel toxins, further enhancing the effectiveness of your detox protocol.

By following the heavy metal detox protocol, you empower your body to cleanse itself of harmful toxins, improve organ function, and boost your overall health and energy levels. This holistic approach not only removes heavy metals but also strengthens your immune system, supports hormonal balance, and enhances neurological and cardiovascular health. Embrace the power of these natural supplements and structured protocols to achieve a cleaner, healthier body and a more vibrant, energetic you. Take control of your health through heavy metal detoxification and experience the profound benefits of a purified, resilient body ready to support a vibrant and energetic life.

Fulvic Acid and Humic Acid

Fulvic acid and humic acid are organic compounds found in ancient soil deposits, formed through the natural decomposition of plant matter over thousands of years. These substances are rich in trace minerals, carbon structures, and antioxidant compounds that play a unique role in both detoxification and nutrient absorption. In the context of heavy metal detoxification, fulvic and humic acids act as natural chelating agents that can bind to free-floating heavy metals, escorting them safely out of the body through the kidneys and digestive tract.

What sets fulvic acid apart is its dual action: it not only binds to toxins, but also helps transport nutrients into cells. Because fulvic acid is small enough to pass through cell membranes, it supports cellular health by enhancing mineral uptake, supporting mitochondrial function, and reducing oxidative stress. This makes it especially valuable in detox protocols aimed at restoring energy and metabolic balance. Humic acid, which has a larger molecular structure, tends to remain in the gut and acts more like a sponge, absorbing toxins before they can enter the bloodstream.

Fulvic and humic acids are often used together, as they complement each other's actions, fulvic acid working inside cells and humic acid acting in the digestive tract. These compounds are typically taken in liquid drops or powder form, either on their own or blended with trace minerals. Many users report improved clarity, digestion, and energy while using fulvic and humic acids as part of a broader detox plan. As naturally occurring detoxifiers and antioxidant-rich compounds, they offer an integrative approach to reducing toxic burden while supporting overall vitality.

Customer-Reported Zeolite Tincture for Kids Benefits

Zeolite tincture, often enhanced with supportive nutrients like vitamin B12 and D3, has emerged as a widely discussed option among parents seeking a gentle, natural way to support their children's detoxification needs. While not a treatment or cure for any specific condition, this liquid mineral-based formula is reported by many families to be a helpful addition to routines aimed at reducing environmental and dietary toxin burden, especially for children with developmental delays, speech challenges, or behavioral sensitivities. With an average customer rating of 4.2 out of 5 stars, the feedback suggests a broad pattern of perceived benefits ranging from improved communication and energy to more stable moods and increased responsiveness.

Use Case Patterns Observed

Among the thousands of reviews we analyzed, a majority came from parents of young children navigating challenges such as speech delay, limited social engagement, low energy, or behavioral fluctuations. The most common motivation for using Zeolite tincture was to gently assist with heavy metal detoxification, especially when environmental or dietary exposure was suspected. This included children with elevated blood lead levels, a history of early medical interventions, or dietary limitations that made nutrient absorption a concern.

A significant subset of users reported trying the tincture during a waiting period for speech therapy services or alongside other developmental support efforts. Some began with cautious dosing, monitoring for sensitivity, and gradually increased to a regular schedule. In several cases, parents chose this supplement after feeling they had exhausted other options. Others noted that they started using Zeolite for themselves first and decided to introduce it to their children only after personally observing positive effects.

The formula's liquid format made it easier to administer to toddlers and young children, often by mixing it into water or juice. The most commonly cited results involved improvements in language development, mood stability, interaction, and general well-being within days to weeks of starting use.

Feedback Insights

Across reviews, parents expressed deep emotional responses to the changes they observed, often describing their experiences as unexpected, heartwarming, and even transformative. Many wrote with surprise and relief, sharing that their previously nonverbal or minimally verbal children began attempting new words, singing songs, or using fuller sentences for the first time. One mother recalled crying in the car after hearing her child try to speak for the first time. Others mentioned that teachers, therapists, or caregivers noticed sudden progress, asking what had changed in the child's routine.

Several reviewers described their children becoming more affectionate, making greater eye contact, and participating more actively in daily life. These shifts in social and emotional connection were deeply meaningful to caregivers who had been seeking signs of progress. Many emphasized how grateful they felt, often using phrases like "life-changing," "a blessing," or "thankful every day." One parent said the supplement made them feel like they had finally "met their real child."

In addition to emotional and cognitive changes, some parents also reported visible improvements in physical health, such as reduced under-eye darkness, smoother digestion, better appetite, and clearer skin. A few mentioned that their children seemed more energetic in the morning, were sleeping more peacefully, or were less prone to meltdowns or sensory overload.

Parents frequently acknowledged the importance of starting slowly, observing responses carefully, and consulting with a healthcare provider when needed. While most did not attribute the changes solely to the tincture, many felt that it played a significant role in their children's improvement, especially when used as part of a thoughtful, supportive routine.

Together, these real-world experiences illustrate how Zeolite tincture is being used not just as a supplement, but as a hopeful tool in families' broader journeys toward supporting their children's growth and well-being.

Most Reported Benefits from Review Analysis

Zeolite tincture has gained attention as a gentle, easy-to-administer supplement used by parents seeking additional support for their children's detoxification and developmental wellness. While not a treatment or cure for any condition, this liquid mineral formula is often chosen to help reduce toxin exposure from environmental sources such as food, water, and household products. Many parents describe meaningful changes in their children's communication, focus, and overall behavior after adding Zeolite tincture to their routine. With an average satisfaction rating of 4.2 out of 5 stars, user feedback highlights several consistently reported benefits.

The table below summarizes the most frequently mentioned benefits based on an in-depth review of thousands of highly rated customer reviews. These percentages reflect how often a particular benefit appeared among users who described positive experiences. A higher percentage suggests that the benefit was a more common part of those users' outcomes.

Zeolite Tincture for Kids' Top Benefits Reported by Customers

Benefit	%	Explanation
Detox Support	32%	Many parents observed clearer skin, better digestion, and improved energy after starting Zeolite, often attributing these changes to enhanced toxin elimination.
Cognitive & Developmental Support	30%	A large number of parents reported progress in speech, attention span, and overall engagement, especially in children with developmental delays.
Energy & Focus	22%	Children were described as more alert, less fatigued, and better able to participate in learning and play throughout the day.

Benefit	%	Explanation
Sleep Improvement	10%	Some users noted better sleep quality and more consistent sleep routines after starting the supplement.
Immune Boost	6%	A smaller but meaningful group of parents reported that their children seemed to get sick less frequently or recover more easily.

How to Use This Table

This table is based on real-world feedback from parents who rated Zeolite tincture highly and noticed meaningful changes in their children. The percentages represent how often a benefit was mentioned in positive reviews, giving you a practical view of what other families have observed. Keep in mind that each child is different, and individual results may vary based on a variety of factors, including health status, nutrition, dosage, and environment.

This guide is not intended to replace professional medical advice. Always consult with a qualified pediatrician or healthcare provider when introducing a new supplement to your child's routine.

If you're exploring ways to support your child's detox pathways and developmental wellness using a gentle, non-invasive supplement, this chart offers insight into what other families have shared, and may help you make a more informed decision.

Customer-Reported Zeolite Benefits

Customer-Reported Zeolite Benefits

Zeolite powder or capsule supplements have gained a strong following among individuals seeking to cleanse their bodies of environmental toxins, heavy metals, and other internal burdens. With an impressive overall satisfaction rating of 4.6 out of 5 stars, thousands of users report feeling lighter, clearer, and more energized after integrating Zeolite into their wellness routine. Its unique molecular structure is believed to act like a natural filter, helping bind unwanted particles so they can be more easily carried out of the body.

In our analysis of highly rated customer feedback, many people turned to Zeolite during times of persistent fatigue, brain fog, unexplained symptoms, or in the aftermath of mold exposure, metal fillings, or intense health challenges. What stands out is the breadth of experiences, some users noticed clearer skin or improved digestion, while others described feeling calmer, more focused, and more resilient. Many even reported Zeolite becoming a long-term part of their detox protocol, returning to it regularly to support their sense of internal balance and energy.

Use Case Patterns Observed

Across the reviews, five key patterns consistently emerged. Many users began Zeolite after struggling with lingering symptoms they couldn't otherwise resolve, ranging from chronic fatigue, bloating, and mental fog to skin rashes or joint discomfort. Others were looking for natural support following specific toxin exposures such as mercury dental fillings, mold in the home, or chemical-heavy environments.

A significant number of people integrated Zeolite into a larger holistic routine, combining it with hydration, clean eating, or other gentle detox methods. Some users began with very small doses to gauge sensitivity, while others used higher quantities based on their personal tolerance and goals. A surprising number of reviewers also mentioned using Zeolite not just for themselves, but for family members, children, and even pets, often noting positive behavioral or energy changes across the board. For many, Zeolite became a cornerstone of their long-term wellness plan.

Feedback Insights

Emotionally, users shared deep gratitude for the improvements they experienced, often after years of trying different solutions with little relief. Many described their results with words like "life-changing," "miraculous," or "the best detox ever." Several people noted feeling clearer, more themselves, or "like a cloud had lifted." The cognitive and emotional improvements were just as striking as the physical ones, with users expressing surprise at how their mental clarity, energy, and mood noticeably improved after regular use.

There were also consistent mentions of reduced brain fog, better sleep, and smoother digestion. One person noted, "I feel lighter, I think more clearly, my senses are keener, just an overall sense of well-being." Another reported, "After struggling with depression, anxiety, and brain fog for years, this gave me back my clarity and peace of mind." Even users who were skeptical at first often shared they were pleasantly surprised by how quickly they noticed benefits, with several mentioning they never wanted to be without it again.

Some reviewers also described "die-off" or detox symptoms, such as bloating, sleep changes, or temporary fatigue, which resolved after adjusting dosage or increasing water intake. These were generally framed as expected and manageable, especially when accompanied by the sense of progress and cleansing.

Overall, the tone of the reviews was not only positive but often emotional, with users crediting Zeolite for helping them feel like themselves again, more clear-headed, grounded, and capable.

Most Reported Benefits from Review Analysis

Zeolite capsules and powders are widely appreciated for their ability to support full-body detoxification. With a high satisfaction rating of 4.6 out of 5 stars, many users describe Zeolite as a foundational supplement that helped them feel lighter, clearer, and more energized. Its natural binding properties are believed to support the body's ability to flush out heavy metals and other environmental toxins, which can contribute to fatigue, brain fog, and immune challenges.

To better understand how people are using Zeolite and what results they most often experience, we analyzed thousands of highly rated user reviews. The top benefits listed below reflect how frequently each effect was mentioned by customers who had a positive experience with the product. A higher percentage suggests that more users noticed that particular benefit, offering helpful insights for those exploring Zeolite for similar reasons.

Zeolite's Top Benefits Reported by Customers

Benefit	%	Explanation
Detox & Heavy Metal Removal	56%	The most widely reported benefit, users frequently noticed improved elimination of toxins and felt healthier overall.
Energy & Vitality	15%	Many users described feeling more energetic and resilient, with reduced fatigue throughout the day.
Immune Support	11%	A number of people felt their immune defenses became stronger and more consistent.
Mental Clarity & Focus	11%	Several users experienced a clearer mind, reduced brain fog, and better ability to concentrate.

Benefit	%	Explanation
Digestive & Gut Health	7%	Some reported smoother digestion, reduced bloating, and a general improvement in gut comfort.

How to Use This Table

These figures represent patterns observed among customers who reported a noticeable benefit after using Zeolite. While individual responses will vary, a higher percentage indicates a more common experience among users with similar goals. For example, if you're looking to support detoxification or reduce brain fog, the data suggests that many others using Zeolite for those reasons experienced meaningful results.

It's important to remember that Zeolite is most often used as part of a broader wellness routine. Many users also emphasized the importance of hydration, dietary adjustments, and gradual dosage to maximize effectiveness. Whether you're looking to support energy, digestion, or overall clarity, these insights offer a helpful starting point as you consider how Zeolite might fit into your personal health journey.

Lymphatic Detox

Clearing the Body's Natural Drainage System

The lymphatic system is one of the most overlooked yet critical components of the body's detoxification network. Often referred to as the body's drainage system, the lymphatic system is responsible for removing cellular waste, toxins, and excess fluids while transporting immune cells to defend against infections and disease. Unlike the circulatory system, which relies on the heart to pump blood, the lymphatic system does not have its own central pump. Instead, it relies on movement, muscle contractions, and proper hydration to circulate lymph fluid and eliminate waste effectively.

In an ideal state, the lymphatic system continuously flushes toxins, supports immune function, and maintains fluid balance. However, sedentary lifestyles, poor diet, dehydration, chronic stress, and exposure to environmental toxins can cause lymphatic congestion, slowing down the body's ability to detoxify. When the lymphatic system becomes sluggish, toxins accumulate, leading to swelling (edema), chronic inflammation, weakened immunity, skin issues, fatigue, and an increased susceptibility to illness.

A lymphatic detox is designed to stimulate lymph flow, encourage toxin removal, and support immune health. By incorporating natural techniques such as movement, hydration, massage, herbal support, and deep breathing, you can help clear blockages in the lymphatic system and restore its natural function.

A well-functioning lymphatic system not only enhances detoxification but also improves circulation, reduces inflammation, supports healthy skin, and strengthens the body's ability to fight infections. This chapter will explore the importance of lymphatic detoxification, its key benefits, and how to naturally enhance lymphatic flow to optimize health and well-being.

Science-Informed Lymphatic Detox Benefits

The lymphatic system is a crucial yet often neglected part of the body's detoxification process. It serves as the body's natural drainage network, responsible for removing cellular waste, toxins, and excess fluids while supporting immune function. Unlike the circulatory system, which relies on the heart to pump blood, the lymphatic system depends on movement, muscle contractions, hydration, and deep breathing to circulate lymph fluid and clear out harmful substances. When the lymphatic system becomes sluggish due to sedentary lifestyles, poor diet, dehydration, chronic stress, or toxin overload, the body struggles to eliminate waste efficiently. This can lead to symptoms such as swelling, persistent fatigue, brain fog, chronic inflammation, and a weakened immune response. Below are the key benefits of lymphatic detoxification and how it contributes to overall health.

Enhances Detoxification and Waste Removal

The lymphatic system plays a critical role in detoxification by transporting metabolic waste, environmental toxins, and excess proteins out of the tissues and into the bloodstream, where they can be eliminated through the liver and kidneys. When the lymphatic system is congested, toxins accumulate in the body, leading to chronic inflammation, bloating, skin problems, and fatigue. A well-functioning lymphatic system ensures continuous removal of waste, helping the body maintain balance and optimal health.

Reduces Swelling, Puffiness, and Water Retention

Lymph fluid carries excess waste, proteins, and fluids from tissues back into circulation, preventing fluid buildup in the body. When the lymphatic system becomes sluggish, it can result in swollen lymph nodes, puffiness in the face and limbs, and overall water retention. Lymphatic detoxification, through movement, hydration, and massage techniques like lymphatic drainage therapy, helps to reduce fluid retention, improve circulation, and alleviate swelling, leading to a lighter, more energized feeling.

Supports Immune System Function

The lymphatic system is an essential component of the immune system, housing and transporting white blood cells (lymphocytes) that fight infections and destroy harmful pathogens. When the lymphatic system is congested, immune function weakens, increasing susceptibility to colds, infections, and inflammatory conditions. A lymphatic detox helps stimulate lymphatic circulation, allowing immune cells to move freely and respond effectively to invaders, resulting in a stronger defense against illnesses.

Improves Energy Levels and Reduces Fatigue

A sluggish lymphatic system can cause toxin buildup and fluid stagnation, leading to chronic fatigue, muscle aches, and sluggishness. The lymphatic system plays a role in cellular energy production by removing waste that slows down metabolism and cellular function. By stimulating lymphatic flow, the body can flush out accumulated toxins, enhance nutrient delivery, and improve oxygen circulation, resulting in increased energy, improved stamina, and mental clarity.

Promotes Healthy, Glowing Skin

Lymphatic detoxification plays a direct role in skin health, as the lymphatic system removes waste products that contribute to acne, dull skin, rashes, and eczema. When the lymphatic system is slow, toxins accumulate under the skin, leading to inflammation, puffiness, and clogged pores. By improving lymphatic circulation, the skin becomes clearer, brighter, and more radiant, reflecting the body's internal health.

Aids in Inflammation Reduction and Joint Pain Relief

Inflammation is often a sign of toxic buildup and lymphatic congestion. A sluggish lymphatic system allows inflammatory compounds to accumulate in the body, contributing to joint pain, stiffness, and inflammatory disorders like arthritis. Lymphatic detoxification helps reduce inflammatory markers, flush out metabolic waste, and improve circulation, leading to less stiffness, reduced swelling, and better mobility.

Enhances Digestion and Gut Health

The lymphatic system plays a key role in the digestive process by transporting dietary fats and absorbing fat-soluble vitamins (A, D, E, and K) in the intestines. When lymphatic circulation is impaired, it can lead to poor fat digestion, bloating, and sluggish metabolism. A well-functioning lymphatic system enhances nutrient absorption, prevents digestive stagnation, and supports a healthy gut microbiome, contributing to better digestion and overall gut health.

Supports Hormonal Balance

The lymphatic system helps eliminate excess hormones, endocrine-disrupting chemicals, and metabolic byproducts from the body. When lymphatic circulation slows, hormone imbalances can occur, leading to PMS symptoms, estrogen dominance, thyroid dysfunction, and mood swings. A healthy lymphatic system ensures that hormones are properly metabolized and excreted, helping maintain hormonal balance and reducing symptoms related to hormonal fluctuations.

By stimulating lymphatic flow through hydration, movement, deep breathing, massage, and herbal support, you can optimize your body's natural detoxification process. Whether you're looking to reduce inflammation, improve immune function, boost energy, or enhance skin health, lymphatic detoxification provides a powerful, science-backed approach to restoring balance and vitality.

Lymphatic Detox Protocol

The lymphatic system is a vital detoxification network responsible for removing toxins, excess fluids, and cellular waste while supporting immune function. Unlike the circulatory system, which has the heart to pump blood, the lymphatic system relies on movement, hydration, and specific herbs to maintain flow. A sluggish lymphatic system can lead to fluid retention, chronic inflammation, brain fog, and weakened immunity, making lymphatic detoxification essential for overall well-being.

A lymphatic detox focuses on stimulating lymph flow naturally rather than using drastic cleanses. The most effective detox methods include herbal support, movement-based techniques, hydration, and self-care practices. Among the most beneficial herbs for lymphatic health are Red Clover, Cleavers, and Burdock Root, which stimulate circulation, reduce congestion, and enhance toxin removal.

Red Clover: Enhancing Lymphatic Circulation

Red clover is a powerful lymphatic cleanser, promoting waste removal and detoxification. It helps clear stagnant lymph fluid, reducing swelling and inflammation while supporting immune function. This herb is also beneficial for hormonal balance, as it aids in the detoxification of excess estrogen and endocrine-disrupting chemicals.

Cleavers: A Gentle Lymphatic Stimulant

Cleavers is one of the most effective herbs for stimulating lymph flow, helping to reduce water retention and support detoxification through urine and sweat. It is particularly useful for relieving swollen lymph nodes and congestion in the skin and lymphatic tissues, making it beneficial for conditions like acne, eczema, and puffiness.

Echinacea: Lymphatic Flow and Immune Support

Echinacea is widely known for immune health, but it also supports the lymphatic system—helping the body clear waste and maintain healthy circulation. Traditionally used in herbal medicine, it promotes lymphatic drainage and assists in reducing occasional swelling or congestion.

Its active compounds, including alkamides and polysaccharides, are believed to stimulate immune cells that help transport toxins and cellular debris out of tissues. This makes Echinacea a helpful addition to lymphatic detox protocols, especially when used alongside herbs like red root or cleavers.

Often used during seasonal transitions or immune stress, Echinacea supports natural cleansing and immune resilience. While generally safe for short-term use, those with autoimmune concerns or allergies to the daisy family should consult a practitioner before use.

By supporting healthy lymph flow, Echinacea offers a gentle and effective way to aid detoxification and overall vitality.

Burdock Root: Blood and Lymph Purifier

Burdock root is a potent blood and lymph cleanser, known for its ability to support liver detoxification and promote toxin elimination through the lymphatic system. It contains antioxidants that protect cells from oxidative stress caused by toxin buildup and reduces inflammation throughout the body.

Lymphatic Detox Support Beyond Individual Herbs

Many lymphatic detox supplements combine Red Clover, Cleavers, Burdock Root, and additional herbs like Echinacea and Astragalus to enhance detoxification. These blends help ensure that lymph fluid moves efficiently, reducing stagnation and supporting immune function.

Non-Herb-Based Lymphatic Detox Strategies

In addition to herbal support, lifestyle strategies play a crucial role in stimulating lymph flow. Jumping or rebounding (bouncing on a mini-trampoline) creates a natural pumping effect that enhances circulation. Dry brushing exfoliates the skin while promoting lymphatic movement, and lymphatic massage helps drain stagnant lymph fluid. Staying hydrated with filtered water and using contrast showers (alternating hot and cold water) further encourages fluid movement and toxin elimination.

Instead of following a rigid protocol, incorporating lymph-supporting herbs and lifestyle practices regularly ensures that toxins are efficiently eliminated and immune function remains strong. A well-functioning lymphatic system is key to vitality, clear skin, and long-term wellness.

Customer-Reported Lymphatic Detox Benefits

Lymphatic detox supplements have become a powerful choice for individuals seeking to support their body's natural detoxification and drainage processes. With an average customer rating of 4.3 out of 5, users frequently describe noticeable improvements in swelling, energy, and lymph node comfort, often within the first few days of use. Many reviewers shared that they had struggled with persistent puffiness, unexplained inflammation, or lymph congestion for months or even years, trying multiple solutions with little success. The results reported in verified reviews suggest that when taken consistently and paired with hydration and gentle movement, lymphatic detox formulas may offer significant relief and revitalization. Whether used for general cleansing, post-surgical recovery, or to support immune resilience, many customers found this approach to be a turning point in their wellness routine.

Use Case Patterns Observed

Most users turn to lymphatic detox supplements when experiencing symptoms of fluid retention, puffiness in the face or limbs, or swollen lymph nodes that did not respond to conventional treatments. Some began using these drops after surgery (including cosmetic procedures like lipo or tummy tuck), while others sought them out due to chronic swelling from conditions like hypothyroidism, autoimmune concerns, or viral recovery. A notable number of parents reported using lymphatic support for their children following episodes of prolonged lymph node swelling or unexplained immune responses. Some reviewers used these drops as part of a broader wellness or detox regimen, especially when addressing adrenal fatigue, kidney support, or digestive sluggishness. Others simply wanted a proactive way to reduce systemic inflammation and support daily drainage.

Feedback Insights

The emotional responses from users were powerful and consistent: a sense of relief, gratitude, and renewed hope. Many expressed amazement at how quickly they noticed changes, with phrases like "felt results in hours," "pain gone overnight," and "down 10 pounds of fluid in two days." Reviewers described swelling visibly reducing in their ankles, face, armpits, or neck, and some shared how long-standing lymph node lumps began to shrink for the first time in years. Several mentioned feeling more "comfortable in my own body" or "finally able to relax" after dealing with persistent discomfort. Others noticed indirect benefits, such as improved skin clarity, better digestion, and fewer infections. Even those who experienced initial detox reactions, such as headaches or increased urination, generally felt the benefits were worth the temporary symptoms. Many reviews closed with affirmations like "I will keep this on hand for life" or "one of the most effective natural products I've ever tried." The overall tone reflected not just physical improvement, but a deeper emotional transformation for many users who had felt overlooked or frustrated with traditional options.

Most Reported Benefits from Review Analysis

To understand which benefits are most consistently experienced, we analyzed thousands of verified 4- and 5-star reviews. The percentages below reflect how often each benefit was mentioned by users who reported positive outcomes. A higher percentage suggests a greater likelihood of experiencing that benefit if you are dealing with related concerns.

For example, if over half of all positive reviews mention improved lymphatic drainage and reduced swelling, it suggests this is a core reason why many people continue using these supplements.

Lymphatic Detox's Top Benefits Reported by Customers

Benefit	%	Explanation
Lymphatic Drainage & Swelling Reduction	54%	Most users describe a significant reduction in puffiness, fluid retention, or swollen lymph nodes, often noticing visible changes within days of starting use.
Inflammation & Pain Relief	16%	Many report relief from body aches, joint stiffness, and chronic inflammation, especially in areas like the legs, armpits, or neck.
Detox & Toxin Removal	14%	Users frequently mention feeling lighter, cleaner, or more balanced, often attributing it to enhanced waste elimination.
Immune Support	9%	Some reviewers credit the supplement with helping their bodies stay stronger during times of illness or preventing flare-ups of recurring infections.
Energy & Vitality	7%	Several people noted an improvement in daily energy levels, reporting a greater sense of well-being, improved mood, and reduced fatigue.

How to Use This Table

This table is designed to help you quickly understand which benefits were mentioned most frequently by satisfied users. While individual experiences vary, the higher the percentage, the more commonly that benefit was experienced. If you're considering a lymphatic detox supplement for swelling, fatigue, or immune support, this data can help you identify the areas where others have seen the greatest impact.

These insights provide a meaningful look at how real people are using lymphatic detox supplements and what kinds of improvements they most often report. Whether your goal is to reduce puffiness, feel more energized, or support your immune health, a high-quality lymphatic formula may offer the gentle support your body needs to feel more balanced and clearer.

Kidney Detoxification

Supporting the Body's Natural Filtration System

The kidneys are the body's primary filtration organs, working continuously to remove excess waste, toxins, and fluids from the bloodstream while maintaining electrolyte balance, regulating blood pressure, and supporting hydration. Every day, these vital organs filter nearly 50 gallons of blood, extracting harmful substances and eliminating them through urine. However, modern lifestyles, characterized by processed foods, high sodium intake, dehydration, environmental exposures, and pharmaceutical use, can place a heavy burden on the kidneys, impacting their ability to function efficiently.

When the kidneys become overworked or sluggish, toxins may accumulate in the body, fluid retention can increase, and waste products may build up in the bloodstream. This can lead to symptoms such as fatigue, swelling, lower back discomfort, frequent urinary tract infections (UTIs), kidney stones, and elevated blood pressure. Over time, reduced kidney function may contribute to chronic kidney stress, urinary system imbalances, and metabolic disruptions.

A kidney detox is not about extreme cleansing or fasting. Instead, it focuses on gently supporting kidney function through proper hydration, targeted herbal compounds, and natural strategies that help flush out waste, reduce inflammation, and assist in maintaining the kidneys' natural filtration ability. By giving the kidneys consistent support, many people report improved urinary comfort, better hydration balance, less bloating, and enhanced overall detoxification.

This chapter explores the importance of kidney detoxification, signs that your kidneys may be under stress, and the most effective natural strategies to support kidney health. Through herbal support, lifestyle changes, and simple dietary adjustments, you can help your kidneys perform at their best, optimizing waste removal, maintaining electrolyte stability, and enhancing your body's natural detoxification process.

Science-Backed Kidney Detox Benefits

Enhances Kidney Filtration and Waste Elimination

The kidneys' core function is to filter out metabolic waste, toxins, and excess fluid. When their efficiency is reduced, these substances can accumulate, resulting in bloating, water retention, and increased toxic load. A well-supported kidney detox may enhance glomerular filtration rate (GFR), allowing waste to be processed and cleared more effectively. Supporting this process helps prevent the buildup of toxins that can otherwise impact energy and metabolism.

Helps Prevent Kidney Stones and Urinary Tract Infections (UTIs)

Kidney stones develop when minerals such as calcium, oxalates, or uric acid crystallize due to low hydration or imbalanced diets. A kidney detox encourages the flushing out of these compounds and supports optimal urine pH, which may help reduce the likelihood of stone formation. Improved hydration and urinary flow can also help discourage bacterial buildup, lowering the risk of UTIs and supporting a healthy urinary environment.

Balances Electrolytes and Regulates Blood Pressure

The kidneys help manage critical electrolyte levels, such as sodium, potassium, and magnesium, that influence hydration, nerve signaling, and cardiovascular function. When kidney function slows, electrolyte imbalances may arise, sometimes resulting in high blood pressure, fluid buildup, or muscle cramps. Kidney detox strategies can support natural electrolyte regulation and help maintain healthier blood pressure levels.

Supports Hydration and Reduces Water Retention

Proper kidney function plays an essential role in managing the body's hydration status. When kidneys are not functioning efficiently, excess water can accumulate, leading to symptoms like swollen ankles, puffy eyes, or abdominal bloating. A kidney detox can encourage the release of retained fluids and sodium, helping restore normal hydration balance and improving circulation.

Reduces Inflammation and Oxidative Stress

The kidneys are susceptible to oxidative stress and chronic low-grade inflammation, both of which are associated with long-term kidney decline. Toxin overload, heavy metal exposure, and cellular waste can damage kidney tissues over time. A kidney detox that incorporates antioxidant-rich herbs and nutrients may help reduce inflammation, neutralize free radicals, and support overall renal health.

Enhances Energy Levels and Reduces Fatigue

Kidney stress may contribute to reduced red blood cell production due to impaired erythropoietin (EPO) output, leading to fatigue and brain fog. Additionally, toxin buildup can slow down cellular metabolism. Supporting kidney function may enhance circulation and oxygen delivery, helping to restore energy, clarity, and overall vitality.

Supports Long-Term Kidney Health and Reduces Risk of Chronic Kidney Issues

Chronic kidney stress may develop gradually due to persistent exposure to high blood pressure, inflammation, and waste accumulation. A kidney detox can help minimize these risks by supporting healthy filtration, promoting hydration, and aiding in regular waste elimination. These practices can play a proactive role in maintaining kidney function and preventing long-term complications.

Kidney Detox Protocol

The kidneys are essential for filtering toxins, excess fluids, and metabolic waste from the bloodstream. They also play a central role in maintaining electrolyte balance, regulating blood pressure, and supporting hydration. Every day, these vital organs process approximately 50 gallons of blood, ensuring that harmful substances are efficiently excreted through urine. However, modern factors such as poor diet, dehydration, high sodium intake, heavy metal exposure, and pharmaceutical use can place a heavy burden on the kidneys. Over time, this strain may contribute to fluid retention, elevated blood pressure, kidney stone formation, chronic fatigue, and declining renal function.

A well-supported kidney detox can help enhance filtration efficiency, prevent toxin accumulation, and restore optimal kidney performance. Rather than relying on aggressive cleanses, the focus is on combining targeted herbs, proper hydration, and lifestyle practices that gently nourish and support kidney health.

Chanca Piedra: The "Stone Breaker"

Chanca Piedra, often referred to as the "stone breaker" herb, is one of the most researched natural remedies for kidney stone prevention. It helps relax smooth muscles in the urinary tract, reduce calcium crystallization, and increase urine flow. This makes it particularly valuable for those prone to kidney stones or experiencing mild discomfort from mineral accumulation. In addition to its diuretic effects, Chanca Piedra offers anti-inflammatory and antioxidant benefits that support kidney cell integrity.

Parsley: A Natural Diuretic

Parsley is a well-known kidney-cleansing herb recognized for its ability to promote urine production and assist with fluid elimination. Its diuretic properties help the body flush out waste, reduce water retention, and support overall detoxification. Parsley is also rich in vitamin C and other antioxidants that protect the kidneys from oxidative stress and inflammation, particularly during periods of toxic overload.

Nettle Leaf: A Gentle Kidney Tonic

Nettle leaf is a mineral-rich herb traditionally used to strengthen kidney function. It supports healthy urine flow and helps eliminate uric acid, a compound that can contribute to kidney stones and gout. Nettle's anti-inflammatory properties can soothe irritation in the urinary tract, and its high magnesium and potassium content helps maintain electrolyte balance, an important factor in long-term kidney health.

Dandelion Root: Liver and Kidney Support

Dandelion root is a powerful cleansing herb that supports both liver and kidney function. It acts as a mild diuretic, encouraging the removal of excess fluid and toxins through the urinary tract. Dandelion also promotes bile flow and aids digestion, making it a holistic addition to any detox routine. Its high potassium content helps counteract potential imbalances from increased urination, making it especially supportive during extended kidney detox protocols.

Uva Ursi: Urinary Tract Defender

Uva Ursi, also known as bearberry, has long been used in traditional herbal medicine to support urinary tract health. Its natural compounds, including arbutin, help reduce microbial load in the urinary system, making it useful for those prone to recurring UTIs or bladder discomfort. In the context of kidney detoxification, Uva Ursi helps maintain a clean urinary tract and reduce inflammation that can interfere with optimal kidney function.

Kidney Detox Support Beyond Individual Herbs

Many high-quality kidney detox formulas combine Chanca Piedra, Parsley, Nettle Leaf, Dandelion Root, and Uva Ursi to provide a synergistic cleansing effect. These blends are designed to help flush out toxins, reduce inflammation, protect delicate kidney tissues, and support urinary tract health from multiple angles. When taken consistently and paired with other supportive habits, these herbal combinations can enhance resilience and performance of the kidney system over time.

Customer-Reported Kidney Detox Benefits

Kidney detox supplements are widely praised for their ability to support the body's natural filtration process, particularly in those seeking to improve their creatinine levels, GFR (glomerular filtration rate), or urinary comfort. With an overall customer satisfaction rating of 4.4 out of 5, many users report measurable improvements in their kidney function, increased urinary efficiency, reduced swelling, and a renewed sense of vitality. While individual results vary, these experiences offer powerful insight into how people are integrating kidney detox supplements into their wellness routines, and the benefits they're most commonly noticing.

Use Case Patterns Observed

Many people turn to kidney detox solutions after receiving concerning lab results, such as elevated creatinine levels or declining GFR scores. Some users begin supplementation after kidney stone episodes, chronic urinary discomfort, or persistent back or flank pain that may be associated with kidney stress. Others seek support following long-term use of NSAIDs, antibiotics, or medications known to place a burden on the kidneys.

A notable group of users also incorporates kidney detox products proactively, often due to family history of kidney concerns, aging-related decline in function, or to support overall detoxification. In these cases, users may be seeking to reduce bloating, increase energy, and improve hydration balance. Several reviewers combine kidney supplements with liver detox or lymphatic drainage regimens as part of a broader cleansing strategy.

Whether addressing lab-based concerns or seeking preventive support, users across a wide age range, especially older adults and those managing chronic health stressors, frequently report turning to kidney detox supplements as a foundational tool for improved vitality and internal balance.

Feedback Insights

Many users describe feeling deeply relieved and even emotional upon seeing improvements in their lab results. One individual noted, "My EGFR jumped from 51 to 73 in a month," calling the change "a state of shock, gratefulness and happiness." Others echoed this sentiment, sharing that their creatinine levels had returned to normal ranges, often after being told such improvements were unlikely. One user remarked, "My doctor said restoring function wasn't possible, but here I am, near normal. I'm amazed."

For some, relief came in the form of reduced pain and swelling. Several reviewers commented on disappearing back discomfort, less frequent nighttime urination, or a return to regular urinary patterns after years of disruption. One user shared, "I finally feel like I'm emptying completely after I go," calling it a huge step toward normalcy.

Skin clarity, reduced bloating, and improved energy were recurring themes, with many users attributing these shifts to internal cleansing. Some also noted a feeling of "lightness" and ease. One reviewer, initially skeptical, admitted, "I used to get grainy bits in my urine, now I just feel clean. I wasn't expecting to notice a difference so fast."

While most experiences were positive, a few users did report detox-related symptoms in the early days, such as increased urination, mild nausea, or fatigue, especially when starting at higher doses. These were often described as temporary and part of the body's cleansing response.

Overall, the tone across reviews reflected cautious optimism, quickly replaced by enthusiasm as people began to feel better. Users frequently recommended the product to family members, and many committed to using it long-term as a regular part of their self-care routine. One review summed it up by saying, "This is one supplement I will never stop taking. It gave me back my health."

Most Reported Benefits from Review Analysis

Our analysis of positive customer reviews identifies the benefits that are mentioned most often. These figures reflect the proportion of users who reported specific outcomes during their experience with kidney detox supplements. A higher percentage suggests that if you share similar health goals or challenges, you may be more likely to notice those particular benefits.

For example, when 57 percent of positive reviews mention improved kidney function, it indicates a common pattern among users, many experienced better filtration, more stable lab results, or greater ease in urination after incorporating these supplements into their wellness routine.

Kidney Detox's Top Benefits Reported by Customers

Benefit	%	Explanation
Kidney Function Support	57%	Many users reported better kidney filtration, improved GFR and creatinine scores, and overall healthier urinary output.
Detox & Toxin Removal	18%	Frequently mentioned as helping the body flush out accumulated waste and feel cleaner and lighter.
Inflammation & Pain Relief	15%	Helped reduce kidney-area discomfort, lower back pressure, or inflammation linked to overworked kidneys.

Benefit	%	Explanation
Urinary Health & Bladder Support	9%	Supported better urinary flow, reduced urgency or frequency, and comfort during urination.
Energy & Vitality	2%	Some users experienced more energy and stamina after detoxification support.

How to Use This Table

These percentages are based on patterns observed across thousands of customer reviews. They do not represent guaranteed outcomes, but rather show the most commonly mentioned results among users who had a positive experience.

If you are looking for support with a specific concern, such as improving filtration scores, managing discomfort, or promoting urinary regularity, this table can help guide expectations. While every body is different, understanding which benefits are most often reported can provide confidence in choosing a kidney detox supplement that aligns with your wellness goals.

Candida and Yeast Detox

Promoting Microbial Balance for Your Gut

Candida and yeast overgrowth are common yet often underrecognized concerns that can influence digestion, energy, immune health, and overall well-being. *Candida albicans*, a naturally occurring yeast found in the gut, mouth, and skin, is typically kept in balance by beneficial bacteria and a healthy immune system. However, modern diets high in sugar, refined carbohydrates, processed foods, and frequent antibiotic use can disrupt this balance, allowing Candida to proliferate and trigger a condition known as Candida overgrowth.

When Candida multiplies beyond healthy levels, it can penetrate the intestinal lining, release irritating byproducts, and contribute to systemic inflammation. This imbalance may present as digestive discomfort, persistent sugar cravings, brain fog, skin issues, fatigue, and recurrent yeast-related concerns. If left unaddressed, Candida overgrowth can impair gut health, reduce immune resilience, and contribute to more serious imbalances.

A well-structured Candida and yeast detox aims to address the root of the issue by limiting dietary sugars that feed yeast, replenishing beneficial microbes, and introducing natural compounds with antifungal properties. This approach helps restore microbial harmony, reduce the burden of yeast toxins, and strengthen the integrity of the gut lining. Many people find that this process contributes to improved digestion, mental clarity, immune function, and sustained energy.

In this chapter, we explore the key triggers and symptoms of Candida overgrowth, practical detox methods, and research-supported ingredients that help support a balanced gut microbiome. Whether you are navigating recurrent yeast-related discomfort, ongoing fatigue, or digestive irregularities, addressing yeast imbalances can be a valuable step toward better health and vitality.

Science-Informed Candida and Yeast Detox Benefits

Restores Gut Health and Improves Digestion

Candida overgrowth commonly leads to digestive issues such as gas, bloating, constipation, diarrhea, and occasional reflux. As the yeast ferments carbohydrates in the gut, it produces gases and compounds that irritate the intestinal lining. This can weaken the gut barrier and allow unwanted substances to pass into the bloodstream. A focused detox strategy helps reduce yeast levels, calm gut inflammation, and promote the growth of healthy flora. Many users report easier digestion, less bloating, and more regular elimination after completing a Candida-focused protocol.

Boosts Energy and Reduces Chronic Fatigue

Toxins released by Candida, such as acetaldehyde, can interfere with energy production at the cellular level, leading to symptoms like brain fog, low motivation, and sluggishness. As Candida is brought under control, the body is better able to produce clean energy and eliminate metabolic waste. Many individuals notice a shift in energy, mental clarity, and overall stamina as their system begins to rebalance.

Strengthens the Immune System and Reduces Infections

The majority of the immune system is located in the gut. When Candida disrupts gut integrity, immune defenses may weaken, leading to increased vulnerability to seasonal illness, recurring yeast infections, and inflammatory conditions. By reducing the burden of yeast and repairing the gut barrier, the immune system can function more efficiently. A supported detox process can promote resilience and reduce the likelihood of recurring infections.

Balances Hormones and Reduces Sugar Cravings

Candida overgrowth can indirectly influence hormone levels, particularly in individuals experiencing signs of estrogen dominance. The yeast may produce compounds that mimic estrogen and interfere with hormonal regulation. Additionally, Candida thrives on sugar and can drive strong cravings for refined carbohydrates, creating a feedback loop that worsens symptoms. A structured detox that limits sugar and supports liver and gut function can contribute to hormonal stability and more balanced cravings.

Clears Skin and Reduces Inflammatory Conditions

Skin issues such as acne, rashes, and eczema are frequently associated with Candida overgrowth. Yeast toxins and related inflammation can surface through the skin, especially when elimination pathways are under strain. By reducing yeast levels and supporting detoxification through the liver and kidneys, many individuals report noticeable improvements in skin clarity, tone, and texture.

Supports Weight Management and Reduces Bloating

An overgrowth of yeast can disrupt digestion and lead to fluid retention, sluggish metabolism, and bloating. This may make it more difficult to maintain a healthy weight, even with dietary efforts. Detoxifying Candida helps restore digestive efficiency and supports the metabolic processes that contribute to natural weight balance. Many users feel lighter, less bloated, and more in control of their body's responses to food.

By addressing Candida and yeast imbalances with targeted support and consistent lifestyle adjustments, you can create the foundation for more resilient digestion, clearer thinking, improved energy, and lasting immune balance. This path toward microbial harmony is not about short-term cleansing, but rather a reset that helps the body maintain long-term health from the inside out.

Candida and Yeast Detox Protocol

Candida is a type of yeast that naturally resides in the gut, mouth, and skin. In small amounts, it plays a normal role in supporting digestion and microbial balance. However, when Candida begins to multiply beyond healthy levels, often due to a high-sugar diet, antibiotic use, chronic stress, or a weakened immune system, it can contribute to a wide range of health concerns. These may include digestive discomfort, brain fog, chronic fatigue, bloating, sugar cravings, skin issues, and recurring yeast-related infections.

A well-structured Candida and yeast detox protocol focuses on restoring microbial balance, reducing yeast overgrowth, and strengthening immune defenses. This is achieved through a combination of targeted herbs, dietary changes, and probiotic support.

Caprylic Acid: Potent Yeast Balancing Support

Caprylic acid is a medium-chain fatty acid commonly derived from coconut oil. It is known for its ability to help balance yeast levels in the gut. Research suggests that caprylic acid may work by interfering with the cell membranes of Candida, supporting the breakdown of excessive yeast. It is also valued for its potential to reduce gut inflammation, helping the intestinal lining recover from yeast-related imbalances.

Pau D'Arco: Ancient Botanical Ally

Pau D'Arco is an herbal extract taken from the bark of a South American tree. It contains active compounds called naphthoquinones, which are known to have antifungal and antimicrobial properties. These compounds help limit Candida's ability to thrive and spread. Pau D'Arco also contributes to immune support and has traditionally been used to help manage inflammation in the gut, making it a beneficial component of a comprehensive Candida support strategy.

Oregano Oil: Broad-Spectrum Botanical Defense

Oregano oil is considered one of the most potent natural compounds for addressing microbial imbalances, including excess yeast. It contains carvacrol and thymol, two key components that help disrupt the growth of Candida and other unwanted fungi. In addition to its antifungal properties, oregano oil is often used to support immune function and promote microbial balance throughout the digestive tract.

Candida Detox Support Beyond Individual Herbs

Many modern Candida detox formulas combine Caprylic Acid, Pau D'Arco, Oregano Oil, and probiotic strains into a single supplement for a more comprehensive approach. These blended formulas are designed to support yeast reduction, relieve bloating and gas, and help promote a balanced gut environment. Probiotics play a crucial role in this process by reintroducing beneficial bacteria that naturally compete with Candida and assist in restoring gut health.

Rather than relying on extreme dietary restrictions, a balanced Candida support protocol typically involves a moderate reduction in sugar and refined carbohydrates, combined with the strategic use of yeast-balancing herbs and probiotic-rich foods. Supporting the gut microbiome in this way contributes to better digestion, stronger immune defenses, and improved energy over time.

A well-executed Candida detox can be a valuable step toward restoring internal balance, especially for those experiencing recurring digestive issues, fatigue, or yeast-related symptoms. When used thoughtfully, this protocol supports a healthier, more resilient microbiome and contributes to lasting wellness from the inside out.

The Role of Probiotics in Candida Detox

While antifungal herbs like Caprylic Acid, Pau D'Arco, and Oregano Oil are powerful tools for eliminating Candida overgrowth, it's equally important to rebuild the beneficial microbial population in your gut to prevent recurrence. This is where probiotic supplementation becomes a vital part of the protocol.

Candida thrives when the natural balance of gut flora is disrupted, often due to antibiotics, poor diet, or chronic stress. As antifungals break down excessive yeast, probiotic supplements help repopulate the gut with beneficial bacteria, creating an environment where Candida and other harmful microbes can no longer dominate. Rebalancing your microbiome this way helps restore digestive harmony, reduce inflammation, and improve immune resilience.

Look for high-quality, multi-strain probiotics that include Lactobacillus and Bifidobacterium species, both known for crowding out Candida, strengthening the gut barrier, and supporting healthy immune signaling. Adding probiotics not only accelerates your recovery but also supports long-term prevention by keeping the microbial ecosystem in check.

Together with antifungal herbs and dietary modifications, probiotic supplementation completes a comprehensive Candida detox protocol, targeting the root of imbalance and rebuilding a foundation for sustained digestive, immune, and whole-body health.

The Role of the Candida Diet in Detox and Recovery

In any successful Candida detox protocol, dietary change is not optional, it is foundational. While antifungal herbs work to break down the Candida overgrowth and probiotics restore a healthy microbial balance, your daily food choices either feed or starve the yeast. The Candida diet is designed to deprive yeast of its fuel source, primarily sugar and refined carbohydrates, while nourishing your body with clean, anti-inflammatory, gut-supportive foods.

Candida albicans thrives on sugar and rapidly fermentable carbohydrates. Even natural sugars, fruit juices, alcohol, and refined grains can create the perfect environment for yeast to multiply. During detox, these foods must be minimized or eliminated to cut off Candida's energy supply. In contrast, non-starchy vegetables, clean proteins, healthy fats, and fiber-rich foods support detoxification, reduce inflammation, and promote healing of the gut lining.

A well-structured Candida diet also supports liver function and stabilizes blood sugar, both essential for managing the die-off symptoms that can occur as yeast is eliminated. In addition, foods like garlic, coconut oil, and leafy greens offer natural antifungal properties while helping restore mineral balance and nutrient density.

The Candida diet isn't meant to be forever. It's a therapeutic reset that allows your body to regain balance. Once the overgrowth is under control and gut health is restored, many people can slowly reintroduce previously restricted foods in moderation, guided by their body's response and ongoing symptoms.

Combined with antifungal herbs and high-quality probiotics, the Candida diet plays a central role in a comprehensive detox plan. It helps break the cycle of overgrowth, strengthens immune defenses, and lays the groundwork for long-term digestive and systemic health. When followed with intention, this nutritional approach becomes a catalyst for transformation, bringing clarity, energy, and true wellness from the inside out.

Customer-Reported Candida Detox Benefits

Candida overgrowth is one of those invisible imbalances that quietly disrupt lives. Many users turned to candida detox supplements after experiencing years of confusing symptoms, rashes, fatigue, sugar cravings, bloating, brain fog, and recurring infections, with little help from traditional medical options. The reviews are filled with stories of frustration transformed into hope. For many, these supplements were the beginning of real relief after years of trial and error. With an overall customer satisfaction rating of 4.5 out of 5, it's clear that something in these formulas is helping people feel more like themselves again.

Use Case Patterns Observed

Across the thousands of reviews we analyzed, the majority of users turned to candida detox supplements for one of two reasons: persistent digestive and skin issues, or recurring yeast infections that did not respond to conventional treatments. Many had already tried doctor-prescribed antifungals like Diflucan, only to find that symptoms returned, sometimes worse than before. For others, it was the culmination of years of unexplained fatigue, bloating, and inflammation that finally led them to uncover Candida as a possible root cause.

While some individuals incorporated these supplements as part of a broader anti-yeast protocol, including probiotics, caprylic acid, dietary changes, and herbal antifungals, others relied on them as a standalone option after failing to find relief elsewhere. A significant number of users also reported combining them with probiotic regimens or liver support to help manage die-off symptoms. Interestingly, some long-term users noted using the supplements periodically as a maintenance tool, especially following sugar-rich periods like holidays or vacations.

The reviews revealed strong patterns among those managing chronic yeast infections, skin rashes, candida-related fatigue, digestive sluggishness, and sugar cravings. Many women shared their experiences with recurring vaginal yeast infections, while others found relief from long-standing thrush, rosacea, or digestive problems that had resisted resolution for years. Notably, several users with autoimmune challenges or hormone imbalances saw significant improvements in mood, clarity, and daily energy.

Feedback Insights

The emotional tone of the reviews is one of deep gratitude, mixed with surprise. Many users expressed how shocked they were to see long-standing symptoms improve, sometimes within days. One user called it "a life saver" after years of misdiagnosis, while another said it "cleared up a problem I didn't even know was related to Candida." People described experiencing relief from bloating and skin flare-ups, better digestion, and a lifting of brain fog that had followed them for years.

For many, the most empowering shift was the reduction of sugar cravings and the unexpected emotional clarity that followed. One user, after years of struggling with fatigue and depression, noted that "I finally feel like myself again." Another spoke of "a miracle" after seeing a chronic rash resolve completely. Reviewers who had tried "everything else" often said these supplements were the first thing that made a real difference.

Despite initial skepticism, many described being pleasantly surprised. Some detailed their die-off reactions, temporary fatigue, breakouts, or headaches, as a sign that the supplement was working. While this was uncomfortable for a few, it was often seen as confirmation that the product was doing its job. A few long-time sufferers shared how emotional it was to finally feel relief, even calling the experience "life-changing."

Among the most powerful stories were those from people who had tried for years to heal using conventional medicine without success. The discovery that something as simple as a supplement could help restore balance left many feeling both hopeful and determined to maintain their progress. "This is something I'll never stop taking," wrote one user, echoing the sentiments of many others who found lasting change through consistent use and complementary lifestyle shifts.

Most Reported Benefits from Review Analysis

Candida detox supplements have earned high praise for their ability to help control yeast overgrowth, ease digestive discomfort, and support overall wellness. With an average customer satisfaction rating of 4.5 out of 5, many individuals shared noticeable improvements in gut balance, clearer skin, greater energy, and a stronger sense of vitality. Our review analysis highlights which benefits were mentioned most often in positive customer experiences.

The table below reflects how frequently each benefit appeared among users who reported favorable outcomes. These percentages do not guarantee results, but they do provide a real-world snapshot of what many people experienced. For example, if 48 percent of satisfied users mentioned better control of yeast and fungal overgrowth, it may suggest that this supplement could offer similar support for those facing related concerns.

Candida Detox's Top Benefits Reported by Customers

Benefit	%	Explanation
Yeast & Candida Overgrowth Control	48%	Many users report successfully reducing fungal overgrowth and restoring gut balance.
Digestive & Gut Health	21%	Users often describe improved digestion, less bloating, and relief from stomach discomfort.
Immune Support	17%	Helps support immune resilience by promoting a healthier gut environment.
Skin Health	11%	Clearer skin, fewer breakouts, and less irritation were reported by many users.

Benefit	%	Explanation
Energy & Vitality	4%	Some users noticed a boost in energy, improved mood, and reduced fatigue.

How to Use This Table

This table is meant to help you better understand the types of benefits others have reported most often after using candida detox supplements. If your goals align with the top categories, such as improving digestion, supporting immune health, or managing yeast-related issues, this may indicate a stronger potential for similar experiences. Of course, individual results can vary depending on your overall health, diet, and consistency of use.

Many reviewers also emphasized the importance of dietary changes and probiotic support in achieving the best results. While supplements are not a cure or guaranteed solution, a thoughtfully chosen candida detox formula can play a valuable role in supporting balance, wellness, and improved daily comfort.

Understanding the Detox Experience

Embarking on a detoxification journey is a transformative step toward enhancing your overall health and well-being. Detoxing isn't merely about eliminating toxins; it's a comprehensive process that triggers significant physiological changes as your body works diligently to cleanse itself. Recognizing and preparing for potential detox reactions and the die-off effect can help you navigate this journey smoothly, ensuring you achieve the best possible outcomes. Not everyone will experience detox reactions or die-off effect, but you need to understand and be prepared for it.

What to Expect During Detoxification

Detoxification supports your body's natural ability to eliminate toxins and restore balance, but undergoing a detox regimen can bring about a variety of physical and emotional changes. These changes are a normal part of the detox process and can vary in intensity and duration depending on the type and extent of detoxification you undertake.

The detox process typically unfolds in three key phases. The Initiation Phase marks the beginning of your detox journey, where your body starts to release stored toxins. During this stage, you might notice subtle changes such as a slight increase in energy or minor improvements in digestion. As detox progresses, you enter the Transformation Phase, where your body ramps up its efforts to eliminate toxins, leading to more noticeable detox reactions. This is when you might experience more significant symptoms as your body works harder to cleanse itself. Finally, in the Maintenance Phase, your body achieves a balanced state with reduced toxin levels, allowing you to experience sustained health benefits and a renewed sense of vitality.

Common Detox Reactions

As your body detoxifies, it's normal to experience temporary symptoms known as detox reactions. These reactions are indicators that your detox is working, but they can sometimes be uncomfortable. Common detox symptoms include headaches, often caused by the release of toxins. Fatigue is another frequent symptom, as your body expends energy to eliminate toxins, leading to feelings of tiredness. You might also experience irritability, and mood swings due to hormonal fluctuations and nutrient deficiencies during detox.

Digestive changes are common as well, with some people experiencing constipation, diarrhea, bloating, or gas as their digestive system adjusts. Skin breakouts can occur as toxins are expelled through the skin, resulting in acne, rashes, or other skin issues. Additionally, flu-like symptoms such as muscle aches, chills, and a general sense of malaise may arise as your body works to cleanse itself. Increased cravings for sugar, caffeine, or unhealthy foods are also typical as your body adjusts to a cleaner diet, signaling a shift towards healthier eating habits.

Understanding Die-Off Effect (Herxheimer Response)

Sometimes, detoxification can lead to a more intense reaction known as the die-off effect or Herxheimer reaction. This occurs when pathogens like parasites, bacteria, or fungi are killed off rapidly during detox, releasing toxins into your system faster than your body can eliminate them. This can lead to intensified detox symptoms, making the detox process feel more challenging.

Signs of the die-off effect include increased fatigue, where sudden and severe tiredness can leave you feeling drained. Headaches may become more severe, often accompanied by neck stiffness, and you might experience temporary spikes in body temperature, leading to fever and chills. Flu-like symptoms such as enhanced muscle aches, joint pain, and general discomfort are also common. Additionally, you may notice worsening skin issues, including increased acne or rashes, as toxins are expelled through the skin. Nausea and digestive distress, such as feeling queasy or experiencing stomach pain, can occur as toxins pass through your digestive system.

Preparing for Detox Reactions

Proper preparation can significantly reduce the severity of detox reactions and help you manage them effectively. Here are essential steps to prepare your body and mind for the detox process:

Gradual Introduction: Start your detox journey slowly by beginning with mild detox protocols and gradually increasing intensity. This allows your body to adjust without becoming overwhelmed. Implement dietary changes and supplements one at a time to identify any adverse reactions and allow your body to adapt smoothly.

Stay Hydrated: Increasing your water intake is crucial during detox. Aim for at least 8 glasses of water daily to support toxin elimination through urine, sweat, and feces.

Nutrient-Rich Diet: Focus on a diet rich in whole foods, including fruits, vegetables, whole grains, lean proteins, and healthy fats, to provide essential nutrients for detoxification. Avoid processed foods, sugar, caffeine, alcohol, and artificial additives that can burden your detox system and hinder the cleansing process.

Supportive Supplements: Maintain a healthy gut microbiome by taking probiotics, which support digestion and toxin elimination. Additionally, consume antioxidants to neutralize free radicals released during detox, protecting your cells from oxidative stress.

Mindful Practices: Engage in relaxation techniques like meditation, yoga, or deep breathing to reduce stress and support overall well-being. Ensure you get 7-9 hours of quality sleep each night to facilitate bodily repair and detoxification, allowing your body to recover and rejuvenate effectively.

Handling Detox Reactions

Managing detox reactions effectively can make your detox journey smoother and more comfortable. Here are strategies to handle common detox symptoms and the die-off effect:

Rest and Relaxation: Listen to your body and allow yourself to rest when you feel fatigued. Avoid overexertion and prioritize relaxation to help your body recover. Engage in gentle activities like walking, stretching, or light yoga to keep your body moving without straining it.

Optimize Hydration: Maintain electrolyte balance by incorporating electrolyte-rich drinks such as coconut water or homemade electrolyte solutions to replenish lost minerals. Continue sipping on detoxifying herbal teas to support liver and kidney function, aiding in the efficient elimination of toxins.

Supportive Nutrition: Consume anti-inflammatory foods rich in omega-3 fatty acids, turmeric, and ginger to reduce inflammation and support healing. Maintain adequate fiber intake to promote regular bowel movements and toxin elimination, ensuring your digestive system functions optimally.

Supplementation: Consider taking activated charcoal to bind excess toxins in the digestive tract but consult a healthcare professional before use. Incorporate adaptogenic herbs like ashwagandha and rhodiola to support adrenal function and reduce stress, helping your body cope with the demands of detoxification.

Professional Support: If detox symptoms become severe or unmanageable, seek guidance from a healthcare professional or a certified detox practitioner. Consider working with a detox coach who can provide personalized strategies and support throughout your detox journey, ensuring you stay on track and address any challenges that arise.

Conclusion: Embrace the Detox Experience with Confidence

Detoxification is a powerful and transformative process that can significantly enhance your health and vitality. By understanding the potential detox reactions and the die-off effect, and by preparing and managing these responses effectively, you can navigate your detox journey with confidence and achieve lasting wellness. Remember to listen to your body, seek professional support when needed, and adopt supportive habits to maximize the benefits of detoxification. Embrace this journey as a profound step toward a cleaner, healthier, and more vibrant life.

Detox for Everyday Health Goals

Earlier chapters introduced each detox protocol individually, highlighting science-informed benefits and user-reported experiences. This chapter takes a different approach: it organizes those insights by wellness goals, making it easier for you to explore which detox strategies are most often used to support specific areas of health such as digestion, skin clarity, immune balance, or energy levels.

The percentages shown next to each protocol reflect data from our *Most Reported Benefits from Review Analysis*, a method that examines real-world customer reviews to identify the most frequently mentioned benefits for each detox solution. These numbers represent how often a particular benefit was mentioned in relation to other effects, offering a practical summary of what users commonly report.

This section is not meant to replace the detailed profiles provided earlier, but to serve as a convenient reference for those looking to match common wellness goals with detox strategies that may be worth exploring. It offers a high-level overview grounded in both scientific understanding and real-world usage patterns.

Please keep in mind that these insights are not medical advice and are not intended to diagnose, treat, or cure any condition. While many individuals report positive experiences, every person's response is unique and may vary depending on factors such as overall health, lifestyle, and consistency of use. No supplement or natural approach guarantees specific results.

This chapter is designed to help you make informed, thoughtful choices on your wellness journey. If you are considering natural detox approaches to support your health, the insights here may serve as a helpful starting point alongside the guidance of a qualified healthcare professional.

Digestive Support

Candida and Yeast Detox (48%) – Yeast & Candida Overgrowth Control. Many users report successfully reducing yeast and fungal overgrowth, restoring gut balance. Scientific support: Controlling Candida overgrowth may help normalize gut flora and reduce intestinal inflammation.

Candida and Yeast Detox (21%) – Digestive & Gut Health. Improves digestion, reduces bloating, and relieves stomach discomfort. Scientific support: Managing excess yeast supports microbiome balance and digestive efficiency.

Colon Detox (21%) – Weight Management. Users experience mild weight loss and a sense of lightness due to enhanced digestion and toxin elimination. Scientific support: Colon cleansing may support healthy metabolism by promoting elimination of waste buildup.

Colon Detox (25%) – Bloating & Gas Relief. Helps reduce bloating, gas, and digestive discomfort, making the stomach feel more at ease. Scientific support: Supporting regular bowel movements can help reduce fermentation and excess gas.

Colon Detox (24%) – Digestive Regularity. Supports regular bowel movements, easing occasional constipation and enhancing gut health. Scientific support: Natural cleansing agents and fiber may help maintain optimal colon function.

Parasite Detox (26%) – Digestive Relief. Alleviates bloating, gas, and stomach discomfort, promoting a balanced gut. Scientific support: Targeting unwanted organisms may ease gastrointestinal discomfort and support microbial balance.

Parasite Detox (31%) – Parasite Removal. Many users report flushing out parasites and feeling lighter and healthier. Scientific support: Certain herbs and natural compounds are known to disrupt and eliminate intestinal parasites.

Urinary Tract Support

Kidney Detox (57%) – Kidney Function Support. Users note better kidney filtration, reduced strain, and overall improved kidney health. Scientific support: A cleaner kidney environment helps remove waste effectively.

Kidney Detox (9%) – Urinary Tract Comfort. Supports urinary wellness, with some users noting improved comfort, flow, and ease of urination. Scientific support: Herbs supporting kidney filtration may help maintain a balanced urinary environment.

Sleep Support

Heavy Metal Detox Kids (10%) – Rest and Relaxation Support. Some parents report that children appear more settled at night and wake feeling more refreshed. Scientific support: Reducing environmental toxin load may support more stable sleep rhythms.

Skin Support

Parasite Detox (11%) – Clearer Skin and Surface Balance. Some users experience improvements in skin clarity and fewer visible blemishes. Scientific support: Lowering parasitic burden may reduce systemic triggers that affect the skin.

Candida and Yeast Detox (11%) – Skin Appearance and Comfort. Many observe healthier-looking skin and relief from occasional irritation or redness. Scientific support: Supporting microbial balance may reduce visible signs of gut-related skin stress.

Cognitive Support

Heavy Metal Detox Kids (30%) – Cognitive and Behavioral Support. Parents describe greater daily engagement, improved attention, and more balanced moods. Scientific support: Reducing environmental heavy metals may help support healthy neurological development.

Heavy Metal Detox (11%) – Mental Clarity and Focus. Users report feeling more alert, focused, and less mentally foggy. Scientific support: Detoxifying neurotoxic substances may support optimal cognitive performance and brain signaling.

Lymphatic Support

Lymphatic Detox (54%) – Lymphatic Flow and Swelling Reduction. Many users observe reduced swelling, less fluid retention, and a lighter feeling in the body. Scientific support: Supporting lymphatic drainage may help clear cellular waste and promote better fluid circulation.

Lymphatic Detox (16%) – Joint and Body Comfort. Helps ease general body tension, occasional stiffness, and feelings of discomfort. Scientific support: A well-functioning lymph system may support the movement of byproducts linked to physical discomfort.

Kidney Detox (15%) – Inflammation and Discomfort Relief. Assists with easing kidney-area discomfort and body tension. Scientific support: Enhanced kidney filtration may help the body expel compounds linked to systemic inflammation.

Liver Support

Liver Detox (58%) – Liver Health and Detox Support. Many users report feeling less bloated, more energized, and experiencing better overall wellness. Scientific support: Nutrients and herbs that support liver enzyme activity may enhance the body's natural detoxification processes.

Immune Support

Parasite Detox (19%) – Whole-Body Resilience Support. Users often describe feeling stronger and more balanced after completing a protocol. Scientific support: Reducing excess parasitic burden may help support immune efficiency.

Candida and Yeast Detox (17%) – Immune Balance and Support. Some users report fewer flare-ups and a greater sense of immune strength. Scientific support: Supporting microbial balance may help reduce strain on immune responses.

Heavy Metal Detox (11%) – Cellular Immune Support. Users describe feeling more resilient and less worn down. Scientific support: Detoxifying heavy metals may support healthy immune cell signaling and response.

Lymphatic Detox (9%) – Immune Circulation Support. Supports a more efficient transport of immune components throughout the body. Scientific support: An unburdened lymph system may help immune cells travel where they are needed more effectively.

Energy & Vitality Support

Heavy Metal Detox for Kids (22%) – Energy and Attention Support. Parents observe that children appear more alert, focused, and active throughout the day. Scientific support: Reducing exposure to certain metals may support cognitive and metabolic function.

Parasite Detox (13%) – Energy Rebound. Users report feeling more energized and less sluggish after using parasite detox supplements. Scientific support: Parasites may compete for nutrients and produce byproducts that contribute to fatigue.

Liver Detox (11%) – Metabolic Energy Boost. Many experience renewed energy and reduced feelings of heaviness after supporting liver function. Scientific support: A well-functioning liver helps clear metabolic waste, freeing up resources for energy production.

Heavy Metal Detox (15%) – Vitality and Stamina. Users report greater stamina and less fatigue after using detox supplements. Scientific support: Lowering toxic metal burden may help restore mitochondrial function and metabolic balance.

Whole Body Cleansing Support

Colon Detox (27%) – Digestive Tract Cleanse. Users feel lighter, more refreshed, and experience a general sense of internal cleanliness. Scientific support: Clearing excess waste may reduce reabsorption of metabolic byproducts.

Liver Detox (13%) – Internal Cleansing Support. Many feel cleaner and more balanced after liver-focused detox support. Scientific support: Enhanced activity in liver detox pathways may improve toxin breakdown and removal.

Heavy Metal Detox for Kids (32%) – Gentle Detoxification Support. Parents report improvements in overall wellness and reduced sluggishness. Scientific support: Natural binders and detox agents may help reduce toxic burden in a child-safe way.

Kidney Detox (18%) – Whole-Body Filtration Support. Users describe feeling lighter and more refreshed after supporting kidney detoxification. Scientific support: Efficient kidney filtration assists in clearing waste and promoting internal balance.

Lymphatic Detox (14%) – Systemic Detox Support. Users feel lighter and more revitalized as their systems clear waste more efficiently. Scientific support: Healthy lymphatic movement is essential for transporting cellular waste out of tissues.

Heavy Metal Detox (57%) – Detox Support and Wellness Gains. Many report feeling healthier and more balanced after detoxifying metals from the body. Scientific support: Chelation or natural detoxifiers may reduce stored metal accumulation that interferes with cellular health.

A Final Word: The Journey to Vibrant Health

As we come to the end of this journey through Detoxification Therapy, it's important to reflect on the simplicity and power of what you've explored. The supplements, strategies, and techniques in this book are designed to fit into daily life with ease. Whether you are seeking to support long-term wellness, feel more balanced, or reduce the burdens of modern living, these natural tools offer support without requiring extreme changes.

In this book, you've discovered how Detoxification Therapy can assist the body's natural systems in staying balanced and resilient. Rather than focusing only on symptoms, this approach encourages support at the foundational level. You've learned about tools that may help maintain healthy liver function, assist with regular elimination, reduce toxic exposures, and promote microbial balance using time-tested and science-informed guidance.

What sets this approach apart is how accessible and manageable it is. You don't need to adopt rigid routines or complicated systems. Detoxification Therapy can be as simple as supporting your body with the right herbs, supplements, and habits. Many people find that these small shifts lead to greater energy, clearer thinking, and more consistent well-being over time.

This book is not just a collection of facts. It is a guide to help you feel empowered in your choices and supported in your process. You now have a framework for exploring natural solutions that align with your needs and goals. With this foundation in place, you are better equipped to make thoughtful decisions that support your health in a sustainable and meaningful way.

As you continue to apply these ideas, remember that wellness is a journey, not a destination. You do not need to be perfect. Small, consistent actions, whether that means choosing a supportive supplement, adjusting your routine, or tuning into how your body feels, can lead to real progress. Trust in the process and give yourself credit for every step forward.

This journey is deeply personal, but it is also shared by many. The *Medicine-Free, Illness-Free Series* was created to walk alongside you, offering reliable insights on Herbal Therapy, Mushroom Therapy, Animal Organ Therapy, Amino Acid Therapy, HOPED Protocol, Grounding Therapy, Diet, Lifestyle and Emotional Well-being, and more. Each book is a tool to support your natural healing process and long-term vitality.

Let this chapter mark a beginning rather than an end. You already have the ability to support your health using natural means. Now, you have the tools and knowledge to take that support further.

Your journey to sustainable, empowered wellness continues today.

To explore more resources or receive personalized guidance, visit AshiHealing.com.

About the Author

Dr. Forest Yin (Jie Yin) is a licensed acupuncturist, herbalist, and Doctor of Acupuncture and Oriental Medicine (DAOM). He serves as a professor and doctoral advisor at the University of East West Medicine (UEWM) and is the founder of Ashi Healing and Acupuncture Inc. With extensive experience in Traditional Chinese Medicine (TCM) and natural health, Dr. Yin integrates a wide range of holistic therapies, forming the foundation of *The Medicine-Free, Illness-Free Series.*

Before devoting his career fully to natural healing, Dr. Yin worked in the high-tech and financial sectors with both large corporations and fast-paced startups. These experiences gave him firsthand insight into the chronic stress and burnout common in modern life. Inspired to seek sustainable strategies for long-term wellness, he turned to the wisdom of nature and the depth of Chinese medicine.

Dr. Yin's clinical experience and ongoing research have helped shape practical wellness protocols that focus on balance, energy, and lifestyle-based health support. His work emphasizes simple, science-informed approaches that align with the body's natural rhythms and support overall resilience.

Driven by a mission to empower others, he created *The Medicine-Free, Illness-Free Series* to share accessible natural strategies that fit seamlessly into busy lives. His approach blends ancient healing principles with modern insight, helping people feel more energized, focused, and in tune with their long-term health goals.

Continue Your Wellness Journey

This book is just the beginning. True wellness is a lifelong journey, and you don't have to walk it alone. The Ashi Healing ecosystem is here to support you every step of the way with personalized guidance, nature-based solutions, and a shared mission: to help more people experience the benefits of natural health.

Personalized Virtual Consultation

If you're ready for expert guidance tailored to your specific needs, you can schedule a private virtual consultation with Dr. Forest Yin at AshiHealing.com. These one-on-one sessions offer a personalized supplement and herbal plan based on your current wellness goals, lifestyle, and health history, helping you create a sustainable path forward using time-tested, natural approaches.

In-Person Consultation and Acupuncture

If you're located in the San Francisco Bay Area, Dr. Yin also provides in-person consultations and acupuncture sessions at the University of East West Medicine (UEWM) campus in Sunnyvale, California, where he also teaches in the doctoral program for Traditional Chinese Medicine. This serene, professional setting offers a welcoming space for personalized care. All visits, virtual or in-person, can be scheduled through AshiHealing.com.

Supplement Recommendation Plans

Each wellness protocol discussed in this book has a corresponding supplement plan available on Fullscript, featuring practitioner-trusted, food-based formulas. These curated plans make it easy to take action without guesswork, offering clear, guided steps for nutritional support.

You can access them directly at:

https://us.fullscript.com/welcome/ashi-healing,

or simply start from AshiHealing.com.

Explore the Complete Book Series

This book is part of *The Medicine-Free, Illness-Free Series*, a 10-book collection designed to help you support your long-term health and vitality through natural methods. Each volume introduces a unique modality—from herbs and mushrooms to detoxification, grounding, amino acids, and more—so you can build your wellness path one step at a time.

Refer to the Series Overview chapter or visit AshiHealing.com to explore the full collection.

Support the Natural Health Movement

If this book has inspired you, and you believe more people should have access to clear, trustworthy information about natural health, consider supporting our mission.

The Ashi Healing Foundation *(AshiHealing.org)* is a nonprofit organization dedicated to public education, natural health awareness, and holistic wellness outreach. Your tax-deductible donation helps expand access to these tools and empowers more individuals to explore safe, evidence-informed approaches to well-being.

To contribute, visit AshiHealing.org and join the movement for a healthier, freer world.

Connect and Stay Inspired

Your healing journey doesn't end here.

Follow **Dr. Forest Yin** for more healing stories, tips, and inspiration:

Instagram, TikTok, YouTube, and X: @DrForestYin

Facebook: @DrForestYin1

LinkedIn: linkedin.com/in/forest-yin

Ready to Take the Next Step?

Scan the QR code below to visit AshiHealing.com, your starting point for virtual consultations, supplement plans, and more resources.

Your journey toward sustainable, natural wellness begins now.

Made in the USA
Monee, IL
05 November 2026

67384065R10083